Sensory Re-education
of the Hand after Stroke

Sensory Re-education of the Hand after Stroke

MARGARET YEKUTIEL

Recanati School for Community Health Professions
Faculty of Health Sciences
Ben-Gurion University of the Negev, Be'er Sheva, Israel

W

WHURR PUBLISHERS
LONDON AND PHILADELPHIA

© 2000 Whurr Publishers
First published 2000 by
Whurr Publishers Ltd
19b Compton Terrace, London N1 2UN, England and
325 Chestnut Street, Philadelphia PA 1906, USA

Reprinted 2002

British Library Cataloguing in Publication Data
A catalogue record for this book is available from the
British Library.

ISBN: 1 86156 169 5

Printed and bound in the UK by Athenaeum Press Ltd,
Gateshead, Tyne & Wear

Contents

Foreword

Feedback is central to all living processes, and control of movement is no exception. Therefore it is surprising how little attention has been paid to sensory function in patients with disturbed motor control after stroke. This book fills a gap in the academic literature on stroke rehabilitation.

Most therapists agree that sensory function is important for motor control; a questionnaire recently sent to therapists belonging to neurological special interest groups showed this. Therapists also agree that sensory function should be assessed though there is less agreement on who does this or how, or on which parts of the body or sensory system should be assessed.

Clinical experience also shows how important accurate sensory feedback is to successful motor function. Most people have tried walking on a leg that has 'fallen asleep' after sitting on a hard seat, and found it difficult. Many people have tried talking after a dental local anaesthetic and found their speech slurred. Anyone who has had a carpal tunnel syndrome will know how difficult it is to hold objects with disturbed sensory feedback.

Sensory loss is common in many diseases affecting the central nervous system such as stroke, multiple sclerosis and head trauma. Disturbed motor function is also common in these conditions. Yet perusal of textbooks or the research literature will reveal little about remediation of sensory deficits after stroke or other damage to the central nervous system. Why? One might argue, not unreasonably, that any functional training approach will inevitably involve sensory retraining and so it is unnecessary to focus specifically on sensation. True, but some physiotherapeutic techniques focus more or less exclusively on motor control. One might also argue that sensory loss is rarely if ever present without motor loss, and that motor function is vital for any movement and that therefore it is reasonable to concentrate on restoring motor function. Again this is a coherent argument.

However we know that after using current treatment techniques many patients continue to have poor function. We should be looking for better treatment methods. Research in monkeys and other animals has shown that intensive specific sensory training can and does lead to major re-organisation within the cerebral cortex, and to changed sensory function. Thus, given the frequency of disturbed sensory function after stroke, the importance of good sensory feedback to successful motor function, the poor results of current specific therapeutic techniques and the evidence in animals that sensory retraining might work, it is important that we start to investigate sensory retraining in a more systematic way.

Margaret Yekutiel published possibly the first and certainly the largest controlled study of sensory retraining. No further studies have been published. She is ideally placed to write on sensory retraining and this book gives us the distillation of her experience over many years. It is an academically sound book, based on evidence wherever this is available. It also gives a detailed description of treatment techniques. Too often therapies are not described in any detail, making it impossible for others to conduct further research or to use the technique in their clinical practice. This book does not fall into that trap. This book will stimulate research into the effects of sensory retraining, and if benefits are found, then patients may experience a better outcome than at present. If so, future generations of patients and therapists will owe Margaret Yekutiel a huge debt for her single-minded and single-handed devotion to exploring the field of sensory function after stroke.

Derick T Wade,
Oxford
March 2000

Preface

Since 1993, when Evelyn Guttman and I published the results of our controlled trial of Sensory Re-education in stroke patients, I have continually been asked for a detailed description of the method, and it was to provide this that I started the book. I soon realized that a 'recipe book' would not do. The subject of sensory perception and its disturbances after stroke is relatively uncharted territory for members of the medical and paramedical professions. To enter into this little-known shadowland of neurology and there try to influence the recovery of the damaged brain seemed to me to need a prior immersion in a vast range of material scattered through the literature of neurology, neurophysiology, psychiatry, psychology and education. I believe it is difficult to achieve the type of sensory-orientated rehabilitation for stroke patients presented here without some familiarity with this literature and with its bearing on the task. This is my justification for the fact that the book is heavy on 'background', so much so that the method of therapy which was originally envisaged as occupying the foreground begins to come into focus only about half way through!

Apart from my gratitude to the long list of writers who provided this background, I have many others to thank. My first debt is to my father, Hugh Cairns, who brought to the house not only his neurosurgical colleagues but also many of his patients over whose convalescence he kept a vigilant and compassionate watch, while we children observed with morbid curiosity their crooked faces, their garbled speech and strange movements. I cannot in fact remember a time before the beginning of what turned out to be a lifelong fascination with the manifestations of brain pathology, and it seems in retrospect only logical that it was children with cerebral palsy who led me away from biology to become a physiotherapist. Nearer to the present time, many passages in the book express my debt to Dr. Wynn Parry for first drawing my attention to the possibility of retraining sensory function. Later, if my growing obsession with sensory matters needed encouragement, this came in good measure from attending an enthralling 'hand clinic' conducted by the late Dr. Eric Moberg in Sweden in 1980. Soon after this, it was the late Professor Marsden who drove home to me the necessity of subjecting any new therapy to scientific trial when I spent a short sabbatical leave in his department. For the controlled trial of Sensory Re-education which finally took place I am eternally grateful to my student, Evelyn Guttman, who carted along her boxes and bags of equipment on some 400 home visits to stroke patients in the hot and dusty – or cold and muddy – desert town of Be'er Sheva. Without her heroic work neither the published trial nor this book would have seen the light of day.

Feeling – like Alice – that a book should have pictures, I originally thought to use photographs of patients, but blacking out their eyes would have concealed an important component of sensory re-education. I thank Janice Shapiro for her pen-and-ink sketches of friends posing as patients: some of them perhaps look too healthy, but in spite of this – or because of it – they add a welcome light touch to the book. My thanks go also to Cecilia Koren for the photography and computerization involved in preparing the illustrations.

Parts of the book were read by Jim Birley, Rosemary Cairns, Ruth Berman, David Yekutiel, William Shone, Yehudit Elkana and Saul Yekutiel, to all of whom I am indebted for good advice and encouragement. My greatest thanks go to my husband who bore gracefully with my preoccupation and supported me throughout.

Chapter 1
Introduction

The progress of medicine has many paradoxical results. We conquer one disease only to be faced with another, and many new treatments bring in their train a host of new problems. The enormous drop in death rates and increase in life expectancy over the last 200 years (Cairns, 1997) have produced not only an alarming population explosion but also increasing numbers of chronic sick and disabled people in the community, particularly among its older members who themselves form an ever growing proportion of the population. The health problems of society can no longer be adequately measured by mortality statistics, but need to be described in terms of 'impairments, disabilities and handicaps' such as the system developed by the World Health Organization (1980) for classifying 'The consequences of disease'. Many formerly fatal diseases can now often be thwarted by various combinations of drugs and surgery, offering the patients additional years of life which would have been unthinkable a generation or two ago. One prime example of this is the great class of cardiovascular diseases which, with no means of treatment, often led to the stroke – or 'apoplexy' – which ended the lives of so many of our forebears. In spite of great advances in the treatment of cardiovascular disease, stroke is still with us, less frequent and less lethal, but leaving in its wake an ever growing number of impaired, disabled people. These stroke survivors may have several years of life ahead of them, but for many of them and for their families the severity of their disabilities and their dependence upon others turn these years into a doubtful boon.

This book grew out of the conviction that stroke patients present a growing challenge to the rehabilitation professions which is not being adequately met. In spite of massive investments of manpower and money in therapy for stroke patients and many studies to assess the value of this enterprise, there is little convincing evidence to show that it is effective. For both economic and humanitarian reasons, attempts need to be made

1

to develop methods of therapy that are more appropriate and more effective for functional recovery after stroke.

There are a number of different methods of therapy currently in use for
stroke patients, all of which converge on the central aim of improving
motor control. An alternative approach is presented here, which focuses
on sensory perception rather than on motor function. The sensory/motor
distinction is not merely a matter of academic physiology. It entails a total
shift in the therapeutic relationship: in the therapist's interaction with the
patient and with his or her brain. Working to enhance the patient's sensory
abilities calls for an approach that is closer to education than to treatment
and which uses the active and interested involvement of the patient rather
than his or her passive submission to handling. The aim is to provoke, not
motor responses or reactions, but curiosity and reasoning and thus the
recuperative powers of the highest aspects of brain function. This
approach, by Sensory Re-education, is well supported by insights from
contemporary neuroscience. It has been shown to reduce the sensory
impairment in the hand after stroke and may perhaps serve as a model for
a more effective style of rehabilitation for stroke patients.

This, in brief, is a synopsis of the case to be presented and argued.
Behind this train of thought there is, however, a wider context – a hidden
agenda – beyond sensory or motor function and beyond stroke. The wider
context is a critical view of the profession to which I belong – with the criticism directed at myself as much as at my colleagues. When I came to
physiotherapy I expected to find a wide field of interest and activity; a
huge area of prevention, treatment, maintenance, advice and caring
reaching to the borders of medicine, nursing, psychology and social work,
but not covered by these professions. Instead, I have seen the profession
increasingly concentrating on the physical apparatus of movement. Even
within this area, in which physiotherapists aim to be experts, movement is
often treated in a fragmented manner, related to specific joints, muscles or
reflexes. Intervention centres on a rather small repertoire of methods
which have been handed down orally, becoming in the process hallowed
dogma rather than hypotheses open to proof or disproof. The methods
use an esoteric terminology and represent some of the best examples of
the mystification of medicine that enlightened physicians have been
inveighing against for decades (Mahler, 1975).

In the process of overspecialization, many physiotherapists seem to
have fenced themselves in from the outer world of people and their aspir-
ations, needs and problems. Bowsher (1993), writing about stroke,
opined that 'the persistent concern of therapists with motor symptoms
may even discourage patients from expressing their views'. The patient is
passive in much of therapy, particularly in the case of stroke; and though

manipulating a passive patient may serve to elicit a reaction or inhibit spasticity, these goals may be quite remote from the felt needs of the patient. Lack of congruence between the aims of therapists and the aims and needs of their patients can be expected to have negative effects on patient compliance and satisfaction, and ultimately on the outcome of treatment.

I believe that the inadequacy of what current physiotherapy has to offer for the rehabilitation of stroke patients is just one symptom – one result – of the direction which physiotherapy has taken in its pursuit of expertise. It is as though we had remained in a Cartesian world, with a big sign saying 'No entry!' over the area of the mind – over sensory perception, emotion, thinking – or with a transection at the level of the red nucleus like one of Sherrington's decerebrate cats. Modern neuroscience has moved beyond the mind–body dichotomy and begun to paint a picture of the 'integrative action of the nervous system' incomparably richer than that which Sherrington (1906) described under that title. Cognition informs even our most 'automatic' daily actions: not only talking and writing, but balancing and walking. Outside the laboratory there are no isolated reflexes or responses. The organism acts and reacts as a whole. When something in the body goes wrong the whole system adapts, with an expertise that the therapist must learn to understand and respect. Even the apathy and lack of cooperation of many patients after stroke – often described as 'learned helplessness' – may be biologically adaptive for avoiding another stroke. Activity in the brain changes when a peripheral nerve is damaged or when we have an arm in plaster, and the changes are dictated not only by the injury but by our subsequent behaviour and its goals. Arm movements are adapted to a sprained ankle, and a stiff shoulder alters one's gait. These and many other examples illustrate the total – or 'global' – character of the body's reaction to injury, whether this is a stroke or a more humdrum mishap. The implication must surely be that we cannot work effectively on only one part of a patient: on one joint, one limb, one 'level' of the nervous system or on the body without the mind.

Physicians and therapists may feel a loss of confidence when they find themselves involved in 'non-professional' issues which lie outside their field of specialization, such as patients' fears and anxieties, their interests and needs. The rewards, however, are great.

Sensory Re-education is presented here, not only for its own value as an intervention with demonstrated beneficial effects, but also as a model for a style of therapy which, being geared to what the patient can do and chooses to do, is interesting and enjoyable and almost custom-made for building up the self-confidence which is the key to rehabilitation.

Chapter 2
The challenge

After a brief overview of the disabling effects of stroke, this chapter argues that the inadequacy of present-day methods of therapy with their concentration on motor control makes it imperative to explore alternative approaches.

Stroke and its aftermath

Stroke, or cerebrovascular accident, has been defined by the World Health Organization as the 'rapidly developed signs of focal or global disturbance of cerebral function, lasting more than 24 hours or leading to death, with no apparent cause other than of vascular origin' (World Health Organization, 1971). These signs are the visible effects of a sudden interruption of the blood supply to some part of the brain as a result of the blockage or rupture of a cerebral blood vessel. The brain is acutely vulnerable to any interruption to its blood supply, and irreversible death of brain tissue ensues rapidly if the circulation is cut off. The clinical picture will reflect the loss of function of the parts of the brain supplied by the affected blood vessel and depends, therefore, on where in the brain the cerebrovascular accident occurs. The most common site is the middle cerebral artery and its branches, which provide the blood supply for a major part of the cerebral hemisphere, and the typical result is paralysis of the opposite side of the body (hemiplegia), loss of sensation in the opposite side and, if the left side of the brain is affected, aphasia. The upper limb tends to be more severely affected than the lower limb, and this is so not only in the case of the middle cerebral artery but for almost every other stroke location except for some branches of the anterior cerebral artery.

Stroke occurs with an annual frequency of around 2 per 1000 people but, because its main underlying cause is cardiovascular disease, its incidence rises sharply with age and passes 10 per 1000, or 1 per cent, by the age of 65. Three-quarters of first strokes occur in people aged 65 and over (Langton Hewer, 1990).

About 30% of the patients die during the first month after stroke, 30% recover sufficiently to be independent in their daily lives, and 40% remain permanently disabled and dependent on assistance (Langton Hewer, 1993). Surveys over the last fifty years show that although the incidence of stroke has decreased (Garraway and Whisnant, 1987), the prevalence of stroke – or the proportion of stroke survivors in the community at any point in time – has increased. This results from the rising proportion of the elderly in the population and from increasing survival after stroke (Klag, Whelton and Seidler, 1989). Over 50% of stroke patients who survive the acute stage are still alive five to seven years later (Garraway, Whisnant and Drury, 1983; Wilkinson et al., 1997) and 20% after fourteen years (Tuomilehto et al., 1995). There has been a gradual increase in both the prevalence of stroke survivors and in the proportion who are seriously disabled and dependent (Garraway et al., 1979). Stroke survivors, in fact, comprise one of the largest categories of chronic disabled people in modern communities.

What is the course of recovery after stroke? Not all of the clinical picture seen immediately after stroke is due to irreversible destruction of brain tissue. Surrounding the focus of destruction are areas with reduced blood supply – the 'ischaemic penumbra' – where the length of time and degree of recovery will depend on the collateral circulation, on the patient's general cardiovascular condition and on medical intervention. Early in stroke there are also clinical signs of dysfunction in areas in the same hemisphere or in the opposite one which, although anatomically remote from the focal cerebral injury, are temporarily incapacitated by it. Both of these are dynamic processes which evolve in the first hours or days, so that the early days after stroke are critical for survival. Twenty to 35% of stroke patients die during the first four weeks, many of them from recurrent stroke (Hankey et al., 1998), the proportion reported depending on whether it is derived from community-based stroke registers or from more severely affected hospital populations.

For the survivors, on the other hand, this period sees a regression of many of the initial effects of stroke, leaving a clearer picture of the residual damage. During the following months the death rate declines, and the majority of patients show improvement in some of the neurological signs and in most aspects of functional disability. Improvement is most rapid in the first two weeks and thereafter progressively slower, so that most of it occurs in the earlier part of the first three months after stroke (Wade, Wood and Langton Hewer, 1985). Clinical improvement after three months has been described as 'marginal' (Kelly-Hayes et al., 1989), except in the case of language which can continue to improve even after six months (Kelly-Hayes, 1990).

Although about 40% of stroke patients who survive the first month recover more or less normal function, the remaining 60% are left with some permanent disability which makes them unable to carry out the basic activities of daily living (ADL) without assistance.

This is the average course of functional recovery after stroke. There are, however, great differences between patients and between different domains of function. In general, the greater the recovery is the earlier it occurs, the converse of this being that in patients who recover less there may still be improvement after three or even six months. If the patient regains urinary continence and the ability to feed independently, this occurs rapidly, whereas independent walking and dressing recover more slowly (Wade, Wood and Langton Hewer, 1985). The outlook for recovery of hand function is particularly poor. The majority of strokes affect the upper limb more than the lower limb, and patients with a severely paralysed hand at outset have both a high risk of mortality and little hope of regaining a useful hand (Parker, Wade and Langton Hewer, 1986; Nakayama et al., 1994). Even if the motor impairment of the upper extremity improves to the same degree as that of the lower extremity, the minimal level of motor function that is sufficient for walking is quite inadequate for normal hand function. For the hand to be used in daily life, a high degree of fine control and discriminative sensation is needed which is seldom recovered after severe stroke and by no means recovered in all less severely affected patients. Wade (1989) states that 'about half of all stroke survivors are left with non-functional arms'.

The effectiveness of therapy

Patients who survive the acute phase of stroke but are still significantly impaired are usually kept in hospital for a period of rehabilitation. The duration of inpatient rehabilitation in Western countries has been reported to average about two months (Shah, 1989). This long period of hospitalization and the special remedial therapies provided make rehabilitation after stroke very costly (Feigenson, 1979; Dergman et al., 1995; Taylor et al., 1996). There is therefore an economic as well as a humanitarian need to establish whether the time is well used.

The effectiveness of rehabilitation after stroke has been the subject of controversy for decades. The question is not only whether rehabilitation is better than no rehabilitation, but which patients are the best candidates, what should this rehabilitation entail, and how intensively and for how long should it be given. It is exceedingly difficult to reach unequivocal answers to any of these questions. In the first place, the period during which rehabilitation is given is also the period of spontaneous recovery, so that the improvements due to nature and those achieved by professional intervention are inextricably confused, and much – but one cannot say how much – of the patient's improvement may be wrongly credited to rehabilitation. The second problem stems from the great heterogeneity of all the subjects to be investigated: namely, the stroke patients, the rehabilitation programmes used, and the areas and levels of outcome evaluated. It is therefore not surprising that studies often yield contradictory results and reach different conclusions. Valid conclusions can be reached only by using some form of random allocation of patients. As it is ethically unacceptable for a randomly chosen group of patients to receive no rehabilitation, the subject has been approached by comparing different types of rehabilitation, such as special stroke units as opposed to general wards, more or less intense regimes, and earlier or later rehabilitation.

From the latest trials, reviews and meta-analyses (Ernst, 1990; Indredavik et al., 1991; Langhorne et al., 1993; Stroke Unit Trialists' Collaboration, 1997; Kwakkel, Kollen and Wagenaar, 1999) there appears to be a general consensus that stroke patients fare better in specialized stroke units than in general hospital wards: their mortality is lower, they reach higher levels of functional independence and are more likely to return home rather than to become institutionalized. This is still not very solid evidence for the efficacy of rehabilitation, but it does suggest that the more rehabilitation, or the more 'specialized' the rehabilitation, the better the outcome. Whether it is possible to infer from this that rehabilitation does help stroke patients recover function is doubtful, since the quality of the rehabilitation provided is not the only difference that exists between specialized rehabilitation units and general hospital wards.

Similar difficulties face the task of evaluating the effects of therapy – of specific methods of physical therapy, occupational therapy or speech therapy, or of therapy in general.

Until about fifty years ago, the attitude of the medical professions to stroke was one of hopelessness and helplessness. Bernard Isaacs described this vividly: 'when I was a medical student, stroke patients were used as teaching subjects when there was nothing else to teach in the ward. They were presented as demonstrations of static neurology ... stroke patients were by-passed on the ward rounds – we walked quickly past the foot of the beds' (Isaacs, 1978). In line with the concept of 'static neurology', rehabilitation consisted in teaching patients to 'cut their losses' and manage their daily lives with the abilities left to them: to get about with a braced leg and some form of walking aid, and to put on their shoes and do up their buttons with their remaining useful hand.

This pessimistic approach to therapy was challenged in the 1950s and 1960s by a number of outstanding therapists who were convinced that it was possible to combat the effects of the neurological damage, whether this was caused by stroke, cerebral palsy or other brain damage. They developed their methods independently, each through a wealth of clinical experience, with a loose reliance on assumptions about motor control and limited reference to earlier research in neurophysiology. They disseminated their methods widely, often many years before getting them down on paper and publishing them. Pre-eminent among them were Knott and Voss (1968), Rood (Goff, 1969), Brunnstrom (1970) and Bobath (1970). Although they can be criticized for propagating dogmatic and unproved therapeutic methods, these pioneers undoubtedly brought about a much needed revolution in therapy for stroke patients, who until then had been regarded as a lost cause. What was new in their approach – and shared by all of them – was that, instead of teaching the patient to use his good side to compensate for the disabilities of the affected side, they focused their treatment on the paralysed side of the body. Their common overall aim was to promote the return of voluntary movement and motor control, and the basic technique in all the methods was the use of skilled handling of the patient to elicit or facilitate motor responses.

These methods have been reviewed by recent authors (Kidd, Lawes and Musa, 1992; Partridge and de Weerdt, 1995; Ashburn, 1995), and only their salient features will be mentioned here. The method developed by Knott and Voss, called Proprioceptive Neuromuscular Facilitation or PNF, uses peripheral stimulation – primarily by manual resistance – to reinforce the patient's maximal efforts to move. Patterns of movement are chosen in line with the primitive mass movements that occur in normal child development. Rood's method also used sensory stimulation – by icing, tapping and stroking as well as by resistance – to elicit motor responses, including postural reactions, according to a developmental sequence. Brunnstrom too believed that recovery must follow a developmental sequence and therefore encouraged primitive mass patterns of movement as a necessary prelude to the recovery of differentiated adult movement. She built on primitive postural reflexes as well as on spinal reflexes. Bobath vehemently opposed the use of abnormal movement patterns as likely to increase spasticity and perpetuate the undesirable influence of primitive postural reflexes. She believed that normal voluntary movement could only appear if normal postural activity was re-established.

The four methods have much in common and are often referred to collectively as neurophysiological or neurodevelopmental approaches. The differences between them however, are not trivial. They relate to the subjects of muscle tone, the postural background of movement, the use of resisted movement and other sensory cues, and the adherence to a developmental sequence. The underlying assumptions about motor control and the different ways of handling the patient remain to the present day the core of both physiotherapy (Ashburn, Partridge and De Souza, 1993) and occupational therapy for stroke patients (Mathiowetz and Bass-Haugen, 1994).

Between 1970 and 1990, some 15 trials of these therapeutic approaches to stroke were published. As in the evaluation of stroke rehabilitation, trials have taken the form of comparisons between the effects of different methods of therapy, the aim being to identify the most effective method for improving motor control rather than to establish whether any of the methods is better than no therapy. None of the trials has produced clear evidence favouring any one method, and there is still little reason to challenge the view that 'there is remarkably little evidence that any procedure improves upon natural recovery' (Wade et al., 1985) and that 'spontaneous neurological recovery is most likely to be responsible for most functional recovery' (Kwakkel, Kollen and Wagenaar, 1999). The trials tended to be too small, thus running the risk of producing false negative results, and the methodology was often poor, but their cumulative weight has led leading physiotherapists today to conclude – although still believing that physiotherapy can help stroke patients - that 'no one approach has yet been able to demonstrate a distinct advantage over any other' (Partridge and de Weerdt, 1995) and 'either it does not matter which treatment approach is used or, if there is an optimal approach, it has not yet been characterized' (Ashburn, 1995). This, as Ernst wrote, 'must be sobering to the followers of one particular school, but it represents the state of the art today' (Ernst, 1990).

With the passage of time, the conceptual differences between the different schools of thought have become somewhat blurred as their adherents have adjusted their theory and their practice to incorporate new ideas, and the different approaches are no longer quite the closed conceptual systems of thirty years ago. It is probably true to say that even if most therapists working with stroke patients see themselves as disciples of one or other school, in practice they are highly eclectic in their choice of treatment techniques (Ashburn, 1995). As a result, it would now be difficult to carry out a study comparing the effects of different treatments, and such studies seem to have dropped out of the literature in the last decade.

If the outcome for the patient is the same whichever regime of therapy is used, the implication is that the recovery of motor control after stroke is not influenced by encouraging or discouraging mass movements, by bombarding the peripheral nervous system with stimuli or by following the developmental sequence of movements. It cannot be concluded that all therapy for stroke patients as it is practised is ineffective, as it is possible that patients are helped by what these different methods share: namely, the prevention of contractures by handling and passive movements, the encouragement and attention of an optimistic therapist, and the like. But it is clear that the whole subject of therapy after stroke needs to be reviewed critically and efforts made to develop more effective methods.

A recent study (Hale and Eales, 1998) raises serious questions about the value of the physiotherapy given to stroke patients. We have said that ethical considerations have ruled out the possibility of comparing outcome with and without therapy. However, there are less fortunate communities in which stroke patients receive minimal rehabilitation or none, so that spontaneous recovery can be studied in a more or less uncontaminated form. One such community is the black, low-income urban population of Soweto near Johannesburg. The inhabitants of Soweto who were the subject of the study had been admitted to hospital with a first stroke in the region of the middle cerebral artery. They were kept in hospital for an average of ten days until medically stable and then discharged to their homes where, three months later, the survivors were followed up and interviewed. Up to now only the findings on their walking ability have been published, but these are striking. At three months, 76% were walking, 65% unassisted, and the majority walking outside as well as indoors. 'At least half ... felt they could walk as far as they needed to', and over one third were able to catch a taxi unassisted. All the patients under 50 years of age were able to walk. These results do not fall below the 65–85% reported in various studies as regaining independent walking after rehabilitation in the West (Hale and Eales, 1998), and these studies refer to walking in hospital. Independent walking out of doors is less often achieved. For instance, only 41% of the 109 stroke patients studied by Hill and colleagues achieved independent outdoor mobility after four months' in-hospital rehabilitation (Hill et al., 1997).

The results of the Soweto study must cast serious doubts on the value of the weeks or months of in-hospital therapy considered beneficial for stroke patients. True, they deal only with the recovery of walking, but this – as the authors point out – seems to be one the goals most desired by stroke patients (Bohannon, Horton and Wikholm, 1991) as well as a major aim of physiotherapy. We await the publication of their findings for the upper limb since, as Wade wrote, 'much effort is expended on trying to increase function in the arm after stroke, but at present there is no thera-peutic approach of proven benefit' (Wade, 1989). The Soweto study, together with the many studies that have failed to demonstrate any differ-ence in outcome between different therapeutic approaches, must lead one to ask: what is wrong, or what is lacking, in present-day therapy for stroke patients?

The neurophysiological methods that we have described address spinal and lower brain centres and are conspicuous in the almost complete absence of any cognitive dimension. They make little or no demands on the patient's mind, on his or her interest, attention and motivation. They are therefore unlikely to set in motion the brain's enormous capacity for functional reorganization in response to behaviourally meaningful challenges that has been discovered in the decades since these stroke therapies were developed.

This is not the first time that the now classical neurophysiological methods of therapy have been challenged, both for their theoretical basis and for their practical outcome. Dissatisfaction with current therapy led, at about the same time, to two additional approaches which should be mentioned here since, in contrast to the four described above, they do not rely on handling but on teaching and thus allow the patient a more active role. These are Petö's Conductive Education and the Motor Relearning Programme developed by Carr and Shepherd. Both emphasize the active involvement of the patient in learning or relearning how to move, where what has to be learned is not motor patterns but the solution to motor problems. The method of Conductive Education, developed in the 1950s by Petö for children with cerebral palsy, has been adapted for adult stroke patients (Cotton and Kinsman, 1983). One 'conductor', instead of a number of different professionals, prescribes a sequence of movements as a strategy for reaching a practical goal, such as standing up, and encourages the patient – more commonly a group of patients – to perform these movements while chanting what is called a 'rhythmic intention', such as 'I stretch my arms forward'. The Motor Relearning Programme (Carr and Shepherd, 1982) also stresses that movement must be relearned, rather than elicited or facilitated as in the neurophysiological therapies. The relearning of motor control after stroke is seen as essentially similar to the acquisition of a motor skill in a healthy subject, and the patient's role is that of active learner rather than passive patient: the patient needs to understand the task and appreciate its goal, to get feedback about his or her performance and to be motivated to practise. The therapist, who functions as a teacher, must understand the biomechanics of the motor task and be able both to analyse the patient's difficulties and to devise modifications of the task which enable the patient to succeed. The aim is to achieve specific real-life movements that can be carried out in a variety of contexts. This therapy draws heavily on knowledge and concepts from the fields of motor learning and biomechanics as well as from contemporary neurophysiology. It is clearly a more cognitively orientated approach to the recovery of movement than any of the other methods of therapy. Both Conductive Education and the Motor Relearning Programme have been used with stroke patients, though not extensively, over the last 15 years but no study of their efficacy seems to have been carried out.

The quest for a different approach

There are thus some six methods of therapy in use, all aiming to improve motor control, but as yet none with convincing evidence of achieving this. As the methods are quite diverse, although the goal is the same, is it possible that the goal is not appropriate? This implies questioning the conceptual framework shared by all the methods of physiotherapy: their restriction to the goal of motor control and their concentration on motor problems. Giving up the immediate goal of motor control and the special techniques of handling used by most therapists for attaining it could bring about the radical change that seems to be needed in stroke therapy. Perhaps the patient – or the patient's brain – is best approached via a domain other than motor control. Since current therapeutic methods were developed, an enormous amount has been discovered about the functional reorganization of the brain in response to meaningful behavioural challenges. In the light of these discoveries (reviewed in Chapter 4), it seems a priori likely that the brain's potential for reorganization could be better harnessed, and the patient's interest and motivation appealed to, through the domain of sensory perception rather than that of motor control: in other words, by using interesting and challenging problems in sensory perception rather than using passive handling and meaningless stimulation aimed at eliciting motor reactions from a passive patient. The type of sensory re-education envisaged here and described in this book could promote neuroplasticity not only in patients with indisputable sensory loss, but also possibly in patients with predominantly motor stroke, with indirect but beneficial effects on motor control.

Sensory loss, from whatever cause, is invisible and can be reported only by the person who has it. It is often overlooked in the examination of the patient. When it is noted, it tends to be seen as an additional sign for elucidating pathology rather than as something to be taken into consideration in the management of the patient and even possibly treated. The examining physician or therapist who overlooks the patient's sensory loss, or makes little of it, is abetted in this by the patient himself who is often unaware that the problem – or part of it – is lack of sensation. This is particularly so in the case of stroke, where a sensory deficit in the vast majority of cases is overshadowed by more conspicuous and more immediately felt afflictions. Inadequate sensation can be a contributory factor – sometimes the critical factor – in poor motor function, especially in the hand. This has been shown in peripheral nerve lesions (Wynn Parry, 1973) and in cerebral palsy (Yekutiel, Jariwala and Stretch, 1994), and in both conditions the functional importance of the sensory deficit was ignored for a long time. As will shortly be seen, a similar situation prevails in stroke.

However, quite apart from sensory loss being one more impairment which incapacitates the patient and an impairment that might be remediable, it is conceivable that one could 'access' the higher centres of the brain and set in motion functional reorganization by approaching through sensory channels, whether this route is damaged or intact. The sensory approach envisaged does not mean bombarding the nervous system with sensory stimuli, like the icing, brushing, passive movements and resistance of current therapy, since these meaningless stimuli are likely to be ignored by higher brain centres as so much 'noise'. The aim must rather be to challenge the brain with interesting sensory problems and provide it with information that it can use. Here it is timely to quote Gregory Bateson's definition of information as 'any difference that makes a difference' (Bateson,1979). A type of sensory therapy is sought which aims to produce in the patient, not motor responses or reactions, but curiosity and reasoning and thus the recuperative capacities of the highest domains of brain function.

A side benefit of sensory therapy is that it must surely be less threatening to the patient than current 'motor' therapy and less likely to provoke spasticity. It is also possible – and this is a great if imponderable advantage – that it may be more interesting and more enjoyable.

Chapter 3
Sensory loss in stroke

In this chapter we review what is known about somatic sensory function after stroke: how frequently and in what way it is affected and with what functional repercussions, what previous attempts have been made to address sensory dysfunction after stroke and with what results.

Sensory testing, and the frequency and types of deficit

The proportion of stroke patients reported to have sensory loss ranges from 11% (Moskowitz, Lightbody and Freitag, 1972) to 85% (Kim and Choi-Kwon, 1996). There is thus a total lack of agreement as to how commonly sensory function is affected by stroke. This is not only because sensory disturbance varies with the location and duration of the stroke, but – and this is probably the main source of the disagreement – because its diagnosis depends on how sensation is tested.

Sensory testing is still in a very crude state. Its development has been bedeviled by the use of a system of classification and nomenclature which Henry Head (1918) long ago described as 'chaotic' and which, according to a more recent appraisal (Dellon, 1988) has improved little since then. The difficulty lies in relating what Head called the 'psychical' qualities of sensations as we experience them to the structures in the peripheral and central nervous system which mediate these sensations. Even in the peripheral nervous system the relation between structure and function is still unclear, but it is nonetheless the classification according to peripheral receptors that has dominated the examination of sensory function since the nineteenth century. Essentially the neurologist tests the patient's sensitivity to the four primary modalities of skin sensation – touch, pain, heat and cold – distinguished by von Frey over a century ago, with the addition of a number of tests (vibration sensitivity, sense of position and movement, and stereognosis) aimed to accommodate sensory function at

14

the spinal and brain levels. That neurologists are not happy with this is clear from a recent textbook of neurology:

> Most neurologists would agree that sensory testing is the most difficult part of the neurologic examination. For one thing, test procedures are relatively crude and inadequate and are unlike natural modes of stimulation with which the patient is familiar.... Embarrassingly often, no objective loss can be demonstrated despite symptoms that indicate the presence of such an abnormality (Adams, Victor and Ropper, 1997).

The word 'objective' in this quotation provides a clue to one aspect of the neurologist's dissatisfaction with sensory testing because, although Brain in his classic textbook (Brain, 1933) uses the heading 'Objective sensory tests' to distinguish them from the 'spontaneous sensations' elicited by questioning the patient, sensory testing cannot by its nature be objective. As the philosopher Gilbert Ryle wrote, 'sensations are not the sort of things that can be observed' (Ryle, 1949). And though the neurologist may perform the tests with great care and record the results punctiliously, the results of the tests come from the patient's inner world and are determined by his or her attention, understanding, concentration, goodwill and a host of other 'subjective' factors that the examiner cannot control. Henry Head was not the only neurologist to cut one of his nerves in order to get direct experience of sensory loss and its recovery (Rivers and Head, 1908).

Not surprisingly, sensory assessments of stroke patients – both by neurologists and by physiotherapists – have been shown to be very unreliable (Tomasello et al., 1982; Lincoln et al., 1991). Even more questionable than their reliability is the validity of the tests used for assessing sensory function after stroke. The tests, as we have said, are essentially those developed by physiologists for studying peripheral receptors. Moberg, although his main concern was with peripheral injuries, inveighed against the standard tests of hand sensation: 'Why should the mere perception of touch or pain by the hand be accepted as a sign of normal sensation, when the perception of light never is identified with a normal capacity to see?' (Moberg, 1964). A similar criticism has been voiced for sensory testing in stroke patients (Wade et al., 1985): just as visual disorders include not only visual field loss, due to defective sensory input, but also the disorders of attention and recognition in visual neglect and visual agnosia, tactile disorders must also be seen to include the 'perceptual' disorders of tactile neglect and agnosia as well as the 'sensory' disorder of defective input. The only possible distinction that can be made between sensation and perception is the (not incontrovertible) one that the former is innate, the latter learned. But in the adult it is impossible to separate sensation from perception ('Sensation ... never takes place in adult life without

Perception also being there' [James, 1890]), and the goal in assessing sensory function in a stroke patient must be to find out what tactile 'sense' – in its widest meaning – he or she has of the outside world and of the inner world of his or her body.

But we are straying into the dark paths of philosophy. The point to be made is that an examination of the peripheral modalities of somatic sensation is unlikely to reveal all the disturbances of discriminative sensation caused by a stroke. Stroke, unlike a peripheral nerve lesion, seldom produces a total loss of sensation in any part of the body or the loss of only one sensory modality. The sensory input relayed by one single pathway from the periphery to the central nervous system is there distributed by a number of routes to various regions – even to some extent to both sides – of the brain, and some sensory function almost always remains. The higher up in the brain the injury, the more likely the result is to be a loss of certain discriminative sensory functions, such as appreciation of the shape, size or weight of objects, rather than the loss of one of von Frey's primary sensations of touch, temperature or pain. If testing is done with cotton wool and a pin, the patient may be reported as having normal sensory function and his or her clumsiness in handling objects attributed to poor motor control when the main cause is disturbed sensory discrimination.

In general, reports of a low prevalence of sensory defects after stroke either do not describe how sensation was assessed – for example, the study that found sensory deficit in only 11% (Moskowitz, Lightbody and Freitag, 1972) – or used only one test, as in the study which reported sensory deficit in 19% of patients based on testing only with a depth sense aesthesiometer (Parker, Wade and Langton Hewer, 1986). When more tests are used, and especially when they are better suited to cerebral sensory functions, stroke patients are found to have a higher frequency of sensory deficits. Kim and Choi-Kwon (1996), for instance, found sensory impairment in 85% of their patients when they used specially designed methods to test point localization, texture discrimination, two-point discrimination, position sense and stereognosis. The patients studied were consecutive hospital admissions, but excluded the most severely affected with whom no communication was possible. They noted that of 25 patients initially diagnosed as having pure motor stroke on the basis of conventional sensory tests only three showed intact sensory discrimination on their tests. As well as using a battery of sensitive tests, these authors evaluated the patients' scores by comparing them with those of healthy age-matched control subjects. Most other studies have used the patient's 'non-affected' hand as the standard of comparison although its sensory function is often disturbed in unilateral stroke (Carmon, 1971; van Ravensberg et al., 1984; Jones, Donaldson and Parkin, 1989; Desrosiers et al., 1996), and this is another reason for the common underestimation of sensory loss after stroke. The report by Kim and Choi-Kwon suggests that sensory disorders in stroke tend to be under-diagnosed by standard methods of sensory testing and that they are much commoner than is usually believed.

Sensory loss can result from a cerebrovascular accident affecting the sensory pathways anywhere from the brainstem to the cortex. In the brain-stem the routes taken by the sensory tracts from the body and from the face dictate that the most characteristic picture is one of dissociated sensory loss, with loss of pain and temperature sensation on the face on the same side as the stroke (ipsilateral) and loss of these modalities – and often others – on the limbs and trunk contralateral to the lesion. Above the brainstem, the sensory picture depends on whether the damage is at the level of the thalamus, at subcortical levels between the thalamus and the cortex or at the cortical level. A lesion affecting the thalamus, on which all the incoming paths converge, is likely to disturb all forms of sensation, sense of position being particularly impaired. The rather rare condition of pure sensory stroke is often caused by thalamic stroke (Kim, 1992). An unpleasant feature of thalamic stroke (though it sometimes occurs after stroke at other sites) is what is known as central post-stroke pain: parallel with the lessening of the sensory impairment the patient begins to show painful overreaction to harmless sensory stimuli and to suffer from persist-ent spontaneous pain over the opposite side of the body.

The ascending pathway from the thalamus to the sensory cortex – the thalamocortical tract – passes initially through the narrow posterior limb of the internal capsule. Stroke here, as in the thalamus, tends to cause severe loss of all types of somatic sensation, but usually without the pain phenomena of the thalamic syndrome. The sensory effects of subcortical lesions further up the pathway, where the thalamocortical fibres fan out, are less wholesale and increasingly cortical in character.

The characteristic sensory impairment after damage to the sensory cortex is a deficit in what is called sensory discrimination. This is a very imprecise term. According to Head (1918), the cortex is not concerned with sensory modalities, but with the recognition of relations in space, the discrimination of degrees of difference (intensity) and the analysis of similarities and differences. Under spatial relations Head distinguished three levels of complexity, the simplest being localization of a point touched, the next level being two-point discrimination, and the most complex being the three-dimensional sense of passive movement and position. The complexity gradient explained why sense of passive movement is the aspect of spatial discrimination most commonly disturbed by a cortical lesion. 'Some loss of power to recognize passive movements ... may be accepted for clinical purposes as a leading sign in the syndrome of cortical disease' (Head, 1918). As regards intensity, the patient may retain a crude sense of touch, heat and cold and pain – and thus 'pass' the standard tests – but be unable to discriminate differences in the intensity or quality of the stimulus. The primary senses are not just blunted, but the patient's interpretation of what he or she feels is confused, hesitant and unreliable. The loss of the third of Head's cortical sensory functions, the analysis of similarities and differences, causes inability to discriminate objects or the qualities of objects, such as shape, size and texture. The majority of patients with cortical sensory disturbance know that there is something in their hand: the problem is to identify the object or even some of its qualities. There may be dissociated loss involving, for instance, the discrimination of the shape but not the size of objects. Since Head's great work on war-wounded patients, examples of such dissociation have been reported in great detail in patients after brain surgery (Roland, 1992), but it also occurs in stroke patients (Reed, Caselli and Farah, 1996).

An additional sign of altered sensory function in cortical lesions is that a very weak stimulus is sometimes detected more readily than a stronger one (Tegner, 1988; Dannenbaum and Dykes, 1990). Another confusing feature is the variability and inconstancy of the patient's responses. They appear to obey no law, 'the patient seems to be untrustworthy' (Head, 1918), and it is easy to make a wrong diagnosis of malingering or hysteria. Head attributed this to a defect of local attention.

It is not always easy to make a distinction between sensory defects and defects of attention. Sensory perception is inextricably dependent not only on attention, but also on memory, language and other cognitive functions, and disturbances at higher levels – either within the domain of somatic sensation or of a more generalized nature – can produce a range of perceptual disorders with or without a primary sensory deficit. Among these disorders at the murky borders of sensory perception are: agnosia, neglect, and anosognosia. They are not uncommon problems in stroke patients, all have an adverse influence on the patients' functional recovery, and they must be borne in mind in any attempt to improve sensation. We shall consider each one briefly.

Tactile agnosia

Stereognosis, or the ability to recognize an object or the shape of an object held in the hand, can be disturbed by damage to the nervous system at any level from the periphery to the cortex. If the lower levels and the primary senses are intact, astereognosis implies a disturbance of higher order integration, and sensory evoked potentials in such cases point to an impairment of 'transactions between parietal areas' (Mauguière, Desmedt and Courjon, 1983). Astereognosis in these cases can be termed 'tactile agnosia', in line with the concept of visual agnosia, a term coined by Freud as a young neurologist to describe a disorder of object recognition not attributable to a sensory defect. It should be noted that it is not always easy to distinguish between tactile agnosia and tactile anomia, or the inability to name the object although it is recognized.

We have described tactile agnosia as though the disorder, although 'upstream' from the level of the primary sensory cortex, is still within the domain of somatic sensation. It is in fact usually, but not always (Feinberg, Rothi and Heilman, 1986), unimodal: the patient has no problem in the visual recognition of objects which he or she fails to recognize by touch. However, a careful follow-up of war veterans with penetrating brain wounds convinced Semmes (1965) of the existence of a non-tactual factor in tactile agnosia: subjects unable to match objects by touch also tended to fail tests of spatial orientation involving the use of a map to circumnavigate objects placed in the room. A 'general spatial factor' in the form of an inability to deal with spatial relations may therefore be involved, which is not specific to somatic sensation.

Neglect

Moving on to the subject of neglect brings us to an even more controversial area. Stroke, especially if it affects the parietal lobe, can lead to any combination of a range of behaviours grouped together under the term 'unilateral neglect': the patient 'neglects' or appears unaware of visual, auditory or tactile stimuli on the side opposite the stroke and this does not seem to be caused by a primary sensory deficit. After a fruitless search for a single basic mechanism underlying neglect, recent research has instead been compiling a growing list of different forms of neglect, as well as a plethora of ways of classifying neglect (Mesulam, 1994). The cases of neglect most frequently described throughout the history of neurology have been those with right-sided lesions and visual neglect of the left side of space (Brain, 1941). These patients characteristically bump into objects to the left of them, leave the food on the left side of their plate and, when asked to copy a drawing, omit details on the left side of the drawing or on the left side of individual objects (Paterson and Zangwill, 1944). Visual field defects, though they are also often present, are not a necessary condition for neglect of visual space.

Visuo-spatial neglect is so dramatic and so fascinating that it has attracted far more interest than neglect in other sensory domains. Visuo-perceptual problems are also extremely common and persistent after stroke and correlate highly with dependence in daily life (Edmans, Towle and Lincoln, 1991). Somatosensory neglect, by contrast, is hardly a recognized concept. It would imply an unawareness of, or a failure to report or respond to, cutaneous stimuli or the position of the limbs, without there necessarily being a primary sensory deficit. And, unlike the visual system, there is no direct way to separate these components of somatosensory perception. The subject has had to be approached indirectly by studying what is called 'extinction' to tactile double simultaneous stimulation. The patient detects a stimulus on his affected side, like a touch on the arm, when only that side is touched, but feels only the touch on the good side if both arms are touched simultaneously. If the arm is touched simultaneously on the two sides of the affected wrist, the touch on the side further from the body is neglected, regardless of whether the wrist is palm down or palm up, indicating that extinction relates to a frame of reference that is defined spatially rather than somatotopically (Moscovitch and Behrmann, 1994). There can be degrees of tactile extinction: for instance, the stimulus on the affected side is detected but less strongly, or wrongly localized, when the other side is also touched. Extinction can also occur when different types of cutaneous stimuli are given simultaneously to the two sides, or when one stimulus is tactile and the other visual (Mattingley et al., 1997). Each of these features of tactile extinction has obvious practical implications for both sensory testing and sensory re-education. On the theoretical side, they suggest that tactile extinction is essentially a disorder of attention, the damaged half of the brain being at a disadvantage when there is competition for attention between the two sides (Kinsbourne, 1977). However, until we fully understand what 'attention' is and how it operates, postulating an unequal competition for attention between left and right seems to be a matter of rephrasing the problem rather than explaining it (Marshall, Halligan and Robertson, 1993). Attention, like many concepts in cognitive psychology, is both invoked as an explanation and itself a subject in need of explanation.

It may be wrong to trace all signs of apparent neglect to some cognitive supra-sensory attentional function. The diagnosis of neglect stipulates that sensation – whether tactile, visual, or other – be intact. That such a situation can exist is supported by the finding of normal somatosensory evoked potentials (SEPs) in three stroke patients with clinical sensory loss and neglect, implying normal sensory input from the hand to the cortex and a disorder above the level of primary sensory processing (Vallar et al., 1991). However, without recording SEPs it is difficult to determine what part neglect plays in poor performance on sensory testing, particularly in patients with such severe sensory loss that they cannot be tested for tactile extinction. And, vice versa, it is also difficult to rule out the possibility of a sensory contribution to neglect. Given the rather slapdash fashion in which somatic sensation is tested and the degree to which sensory loss is undetected, not all patients with somatosensory neglect may have normal sensory function. The uncertainty and variability of head injuried patients' responses to sensory testing which Head described and which he attributed to defective attention could also be caused, or exacerbated, by defects at a lower level of sensory processing: there could be less information available, as well as less efficient integration and processing of this information, all leading to the stimulus being poorly attended to. Tactile extinction can be prevented by stimulating the affected side two or three seconds before the other side (Critchley, 1949), suggesting that sensory processing may take longer on the damaged side of the brain.

Orienting the gaze, with eyes closed or in the dark, towards the stimulated place produces both faster detection of cutaneous stimuli in healthy subjects (Honoré, Bourdeaud'hui and Sparrow, 1989) and a decrease in the incidence of tactile extinction in stroke patients (Larmande and Cambier, 1981). This is a useful piece of information for anyone trying to improve a patient's sensory function. It also underlines the difficulty of separating sensation from attention. We are, after all, continuously bombarded by sensory stimuli, the majority of which never reach consciousness: they become sensations only if we 'attend' to them. It is this process of 'attending to', of sharing, switching and maintaining attention, which is often damaged by stroke, with or without damage to lower levels of the sensory pathways. 'Neglect' is an umbrella term (Driver, 1994) used to describe the severest forms of inattention to the opposite side of the body and space, whereas extinction can probably be regarded as a form of 'mini-neglect'.

Anosognosia

If, with agnosia, the patient fails to recognize objects presented to one of his senses, and, with neglect, the unawareness embraces half his body and/or half of space, with anosognosia he is unaware of his illness or impairment. He may make light of it or deny it altogether. Denial can be highly selective, with the patients aware of their hemiplegia but not of their hemi-blindness, or vice versa (Bisiach et al., 1986). Anosognosia shows no clear association with clinical severity or with the presence of neglect. It has been found in 21% of acute stroke patients, predominantly in those with right hemisphere stroke but with no other association with stroke location (Pedersen et al., 1996).

I cannot leave the subject of neglect and anosognosia without mentioning a fascinating and little known study of 'experimentally induced somatagnosia' in healthy undergraduates published thirty years ago (Sullivan, 1969). With a pencil in their gloved right hand, subjects sat in a poorly lit room in front of a black box containing a two-way mirror and lit either from above or below. They were asked to draw a straight line between two parallel lines marked on a sheet of paper on the bottom of the box. The lighting showed them either their own hand doing this, or, after tilting the viewing slit and changing the illumination, the gloved hand of the hidden experimenter drawing a line on the paper on the back of the box. In many trials, the experimenter drew a line which deviated from the direction which the subject's drawing was taking, thus presenting him or her with a conflict between somatic and visual cues. In judging their own performance, all thirty students ignored the sensory cues from their movements and accepted the visual information as true. Although there was none of the impairment of sensation or motor function of stroke, Sullivan pointed out that they 'often made spontaneous remarks which were similar to those which might be made by stroke patients'. Examples illustrating somatagnosia were: 'My motor coordination is all off...I feel disoriented...my hand is disoriented from me... not part of me', or 'I'm looking at my hand but it doesn't belong to me...I feel spastic'. Others showed explicit verbal denial: 'I drew that line because I wanted to...your definition of straight is ambiguous...I see that as a straight line', and there were also defensive reactions, such as 'the line of vision is too restricting... arm movements are restricted and these silly gloves don't allow you to draw right'. Many also showed signs of great anxiety. Sullivan's experiment provides much food for thought. The students' remarks hint that some of the behaviour of stroke patients described as neglect or anosognosia may be not so much a direct expression of brain pathology as an adaptive reaction to it. Denny-Brown, describing how Kurt Goldstein's organismic (holistic) viewpoint led him to see the brain-injured patient compensating for his difficulties by avoiding potentially upsetting stimuli, quoted Goldstein as saying: 'In order to readjust itself to the world, the injured organism has withdrawn from numerous points of contact with it and has attained a readaptation to a shrunken environment' (Denny-Brown, 1966).

The functional implications of sensory loss

Implicit in the consideration of sensory loss up to this point has been the assumption that it contributes to the stroke patient's disability in daily life. At first glance this seems a reasonable assumption. One's own experience, of how difficult it is to rinse one's mouth after a purely 'sensory' injection at the dentist or to walk when one's leg has 'gone to sleep', provides a compelling demonstration of the disabling effect of disturbed sensation, and the matter seems to need no further proof. However, the relation between sensation and movement is neither direct nor simple. We shall consider first the role of sensation in movement and then the effect of sensory disturbances on the recovery of function after stroke.

Marsden's team of neurophysiologists had the opportunity to make an exhaustive examination of a man 'deafferented' by a severe peripheral neuropathy affecting only the sensory nerves (Rothwell et al., 1982). He had no perception in his hands of position, movement, touch, vibration or pin-prick, and complete inability to judge the size, weight or form of objects placed in his hands. In spite of being able to perform many motor tasks in the laboratory, 'his hands were relatively useless to him in daily life when undertaking fine tasks' (Marsden, Rothwell and Day, 1984), one of his principal problems being an inability to maintain muscle contraction, for instance, for holding a cup or a pen. Recent studies of similar patients have shown that loss of sensation has a particularly disruptive effect on everyday activities which involve co-ordinated movement at the shoulder, elbow and hand (Sainburg. Poizner and Ghez, 1993). Westing and Johansson (1984) point to the crucial importance of cutaneous sensation for maintaining and adjusting the force with which objects are held and the fine safety margin normally achieved against the object slipping. Any blunting of sensation means setting a larger safety margin and using unnecessarily large grip forces. Cope (1991) found that grip forces used by elderly subjects, with thresholds for two-point discrimination four times that of young adults, were twice those of the younger subjects.

What is the effect of sensory loss on motor function in patients with cerebral lesions? Jeannerod was one of the first to study this subject in detail, in a single patient with severe hemianaesthesia due to a cortical lesion in the left parietal lobe (Jeannerod, Michel and Prablanc, 1984). Clinical tests of motor function were all normal, she could make simple movements of one finger, and she could use her right hand to a certain extent in everyday activities as long as she could see it. But without vision the movements of her arm became 'awkward and inefficient'. Reaching and grasping an object were disturbed, and she was unable to maintain a constant level of force. Pause and colleagues found defects of force control, fine movements and manipulation of objects in all of nine patients with sensory deficits after parietal lesions, patients with more posterior parietal lesions having a marked disorder of purposive exploratory movements (Pause et al., 1989). The difficulty which parietal patients have with gripping and manipulating objects has been observed frequently (Motomura et al., 1990; Robertson and Jones, 1994).

It should be noted here that damage to either hemisphere can cause subtle disturbances of both sensory and motor function not only on the contralateral side but also, though less severe, ipsilateral to the lesion (Carmon, 1971; Van Ravensberg et al., 1984; Jones, Donaldson and Parkin,

1989; Desrosiers et al., 1996; Kim and Choi-Kwon, 1996). In spite of this, stroke patients are naturally inclined to do as much as possible with their less affected arm, and this is responsible for what is called 'learned non-use', or the habit of not using the affected extremity even if it has recovered some potential function. This, which was first described by Taub (1980) working with deafferented monkeys, is undoubtedly a factor contributing to the poor recovery of upper limb function after stroke, though not a factor in recovery of the lower limb which has no substitute for standing and walking. A remarkable experiment directed by Wolf showed that it is possible to counteract the effects of learned non-use and improve the function of the affected arm by restraining the patient's 'good' arm in a sling for 8 hours a day for two weeks (Wolf et al., 1989).

The problems in everyday use of the hand caused by parietal lesions and disturbance of sensory perceptual function suggest that sensory loss must have a deleterious influence on functional recovery after stroke. Although this has been borne out by many studies, the functional import-ance of sensory loss is generally underestimated. I trace this in part to a very influential paper by Fugl-Meyer and his colleagues which has been widely read by therapists (Fugl-Meyer et al., 1975). Although only three out of nine patients followed up for one year after stroke had significant sensory loss, these three showed improved voluntary movement of the wrist and hand, and this meagre material led to the conclusion that 'sensory qualities...could be correlated neither to the maximum motor behaviour finally achieved nor to the steepness of the individual's motor development curves'. There have, however, been repeated reports – from larger samples of patients – of the negative effects of sensory loss on functional outcome after stroke. One of the earliest studies (Van Buskirk and Webster, 1955) reported that although stroke patients without sensory loss averaged 68 days in the rehabilitation hospital, the average stay of patients with persistent sensory loss was 236 days and their functional recovery was still unsatisfactory. Anderson (1971), in a follow-up of 271 stroke patients, found that the 30% with persistent sensory defects achieved significantly lower levels of functional independence: patients with additional signs of neglect had even lower achievements. Similar conclusions have been reached by other studies (Stern et al, 1971: Steinberg, 1973; Smith, Akhtar and Garraway, 1983; Hanger and Sainsbury, 1996). Sensory evoked potentials (SEPs), which represent an objective picture of the cortical reception and transmission of sensory input, are predictive of functional recovery after stroke (Kusoffsky, Wadell and Nilsson, 1982; La Joie, Reddy and Melvin, 1982; Chester and McLaren, 1989; Zeman and Yiannikas, 1989).

One of the problems of evaluating the contribution of sensory loss to long-term disability after stroke is that a sensory as well as a motor impairment implies in general a larger area of brain damage, and the greater the neurological damage the worse the outcome. Survivors of acute stroke are more likely to die within a year if they have sensory loss (Sheikh et al., 1983). The relationship with the extent of brain damage is expressed in Reding's classification of stroke according to whether it produces motor deficit only, motor plus somatic sensory deficit, or both of these plus a visual defect, a classification which is highly predictive of functional outcome (Reding, 1990), as well as of length of stay in hospital and discharge destination (Gottlieb et al., 1997). Any additional neglect or anosognosia adds to the likelihood of a poor outcome. For instance, tactile inattention at one month is associated with greater functional impairment at six months (Barer, 1990), and anosognosia has a profound influence on prognosis (Pedersen et al., 1996). Rose found tactile extinction in 50% of patients three weeks after stroke; it was much more common in patients with right hemisphere stroke than in those with left, and it was an important predictor of functional outcome (Rose et al., 1994).

The treatment of sensory loss

Bobath, founder of one of the most widely used methods of stroke therapy, gave first place to sensory disturbance in a list of 'factors interfering with normal motor performance in adult hemiplegia' and recognized that 'the patient with severe and persistent sensory deficit has a poor prognosis for functional recovery' (Bobath, 1970). However she did not offer any suggestions for reducing this deficit. The few attempts that have been made to treat sensory problems in stroke patients have for the most part been initiated outside the therapeutic professions.

The earliest seems to be that of Forster and Shields (1959), two physicians working in rehabilitation in Bethesda. They drew attention to the functionally disabling effect of sensory loss in cerebral lesions, particularly of the parietal lobe, and described a method of sensory re-education focusing on sense of position and the discrimination of weight, size, shape and texture of objects. During much of the therapy, patients worked with their hand in an open box lined with mirrors. Their paper unfortunately includes only one case history, but they state that 'the results to date have been so encouraging that we hope to be able to amplify the therapy'.

Inspired by this, a method for training tactile object recognition was described using mirrors to give three-dimensional feedback (Vinograd, Taylor and Grossman, 1962), but the effects of this training were not investigated systematically. Van Deusen Fox (1964) carried out a controlled trial of the effects of pressure and cutaneous stimulation to the forearm, hand and fingers, and found that this behaviourally meaningless treatment had no significant effect on stereognosis or on the recognition of letters traced on the skin (graphaesthesia).

The next contribution comes from a fourth year medical student in Philadelphia (Goldman, 1966) and deals with the phenomenon of extinction in double simultaneous stimulation (DSS) described earlier in this chapter. In a crossover controlled trial in 20 patients, Goldman showed that DSS perception could be improved and errors reduced by giving daily teaching sessions for two weeks, where 'the teaching process focused attention on one error at a time starting with the simplest task and proceeding to more difficult ones'.

The next essay in sensory re-education after stroke is from the Rehabilitation Centre of Hawaii (Anderson and Choy, 1970). Anderson (1971) has already been cited as among the first to document the negative effect of sensory defects on patients' achievement of functional independence. Recognizing that sensory loss, particularly in parietal strokes, is often accompanied by disorders of space perception and by unilateral neglect of both body and space, Anderson developed a programme of therapy comprising stimulation (by ice, brushes or rough cloths), puzzles and games to foster perception of spatial relations of objects, and, throughout all the therapy, emphasis on encouraging the patient to 'cross the mid-line'. This programme was stated to have 'proven beneficial in allowing patients ... to reach higher levels of independence', and the authors noted that since its introduction the proportion of their stroke patients reaching independence had risen from 64% to 74%.

The cause of sensory-perceptual training had a set-back in 1971 when a small but well designed controlled study of perceptual training, including manual object identification, reported negative results: improvement was no better in the experimental group than in the control group on any of the many measures of outcome used (Taylor et al., 1971).

Later in the 1970s a group in New York explored the possibility of treating the perceptual problems of patients with right hemisphere stroke. After showing in a controlled trial that disorders of visual perception could be lessened by teaching patients to scan the visual environment (Weinberg et al., 1977), they turned their attention to problems of somatic sensory awareness and spatial organization (Weinberg et al., 1979). Sensory training was directed to awareness of both sides of the trunk, tactile location of the mid-line of the body and location – on a model – of points on the back touched by the therapist. Patients given this training showed significant improvement on these tasks, whereas in control patients there was no improvement.

These early studies, meagre as they are, do show that some attention was beginning to be paid to sensory perceptual deficits in stroke and a start made in trying to treat them. In retrospect this can perhaps be seen as an expression of the then relatively new therapeutic attempt to treat neurological impairments. However, instead of leading on to further exploration of the possibilities of sensory re-education, the early studies were followed by a ten-year gap during which interest in the subject seems to have died. By contrast, therapy for cognitive and visuo-perceptual impairments blossomed during this period.

At last, in 1988, Dannenbaum and Dykes recalled the subject from oblivion, in a paper reviewing sensory loss in stroke and its implications for function and proposing a programme of therapy to treat it (Dannenbaum and Dykes, 1988). They stated that 'the goal is to gain a larger cortical representation for those skin surfaces needed to perform daily tasks.' Treatment began with electrical stimulation using a 100-Hz current at an intensity high enough to be felt without causing pain, progressing to stroking with Velcro. In both procedures, the patient attempted to locate the area or finger being stimulated. At a later stage, common utensils of daily life were modified – often by the addition of Velcro – and patients were trained in handling and using them with and without vision. In recognition of the importance of motivation, each patient's training was directed to tasks which he or she felt were important. This very interesting paper mentions an on-going pilot study of the treatment of six patients with severe sensory deficits from one month to ten years after stroke, and describes the slow but definite improvement in both sensation and use of the hand in one of the patients. Apart from the story of this one patient, no study seems to have been published on the effect of this treatment regime, although it was advocated again five years later (Dannenbaum and Jones, 1993).

So far, the record of sensory re-education for stroke patients seems to have been rather like the study of the early hominids – a tooth here, a jaw-bone there, and more speculation than hard facts. However, the subject has gained momentum in the present decade. This is due not only to the work on which this book is based, but also to research by a group in Australia (Carey, Matyas and Oke, 1990; Carey, Matyas and Oke, 1993). Carey (1995) has reviewed the whole subject thoroughly, and she and her colleagues have been developing much needed methods of testing tactile and proprioceptive sensation which are reliable and suited to stroke patients (Carey, Oke and Matyas, 1996). They also reported encouraging results of sensory training in a small number of patients 1–6 months after stroke: in texture discrimination (8 patients) and sense of position at the wrist (4 patients). The main difference between their approach and the one advocated in this book is that, in pursuit of a tight experimental design, they gave their patients 'task specific training', and 'training tasks were the same as the assessment tasks' (Carey, Matyas and Oke, 1993). This had the great advantage of enabling them to define the treatment with a precision that is rare in trials of therapy, but it also meant that the goal of the treatment was in effect restricted to training patients how to pass the tests.

Attempts to treat somatosensory problems in stroke patients have thus been few and far between, and the results not always encouraging. The subject remains an important one which deserves more attention than it has received.

Chapter 4
The theoretical basis of Sensory Re-education

This chapter opens with a description of the sources which inspired and guided the development of Sensory Re-education. The second and third sections present data on neural plasticity in peripheral and central lesions which suggest what mechanisms may be available for sensory recovery. This material provides the guidelines, set out in the fourth section, for developing a method of active intervention to promote sensory recovery after stroke. Evidence that the method of Sensory Re-education is effective is presented later in the book (Chapter 9) after a detailed description of the method.

Sources

We have seen that although somato-sensory deficit is a common and disabling result of stroke, there have been few systematic attempts to restore sensory function and even fewer studies to measure the effectiveness of such intervention. As a result, the method of sensory re-education described in this book has little in the way of direct antecedents. The initial inspiration came from the work of Wynn Parry, described below, which showed that the generally poor level of hand sensation seen in patients after sutured median nerve lesions could be greatly improved by systematic sensory retraining. Sensory loss had long been known to predict a poor functional outcome in both peripheral and central lesions, and it was generally considered untreatable. But now, if a patient with a severed and sutured median nerve could regain the sensory function of his or her hand by 'retraining', couldn't something similar be done for patients with sensory loss as a result of brain damage? A preliminary attempt at sensory retraining in patients with a variety of central lesions (Yekutiel, 1977) led to the gradual elaboration of the method of Sensory Re-education for stroke patients presented here and to a controlled trial which established its validity (Yekutiel and Guttman, 1993).

29

In 1974 I heard Wynn Parry lecture on the rehabilitation programme which he directed at the Royal Air Force centre at Chessington, near London. Wynn Parry described a method of sensory retraining, notably for patients with median nerve lesions, which led to levels of sensory recovery rarely achieved before (Wynn Parry, 1973). Visiting Chessington, I encountered a style of rehabilitation that I had not met before. The patients – airmen and other members of the armed forces – were busy all day with a series of prescribed activities which included not only traditional therapy but also such novel 'treatments' as playing puff-billiards, tiddlywinks, or draughts with pieces of prescribed size and weight. A special programme of formal sensory retraining was started at the first return of sensation to the fingers.

Sensory re-education at Chessington

Patients were tested monthly for localization of touch and recognition of objects. Sensory retraining was given in a number of short sessions throughout the day, using a vast array of objects, materials and games. The first sensory tasks were weight and shape discrimination with wooden blocks held in the hand or placed on the table and palpated. Patients then moved on to texture discrimination, using pieces of sandpaper, velvet and the like, progressing in the final stage to the recognition of common everyday objects. 'Large familiar objects were used at first, such as tennis balls, matchboxes and nail brushes, with a gradual progression to smaller objects as improvement occurred' (Wynn Parry and Salter, 1976). To retain the patient's interest, games appropriate to their level of recovery were prescribed at every stage.

> Objects, or materials of different textures, can be buried in a bowl of sand and the patient asked to search for and identify them. Wooden shapes can be fitted back into their appropriate holes in a board, and the time taken noted, with patients competing against each other. Later, wooden letters are given to the patient who has to form words and anagrams, and leave a message for the therapists (Wynn Parry, 1973).

So much for the sensory tasks. The basic method of retraining was that the patient repeatedly compared what he sensed with his eyes closed with what he saw when he opened his eyes. In this way, he used vision to help him learn to interpret the abnormal sensory input transmitted by the regenerating nerve. This view of the recovery of sensory function as a learning process was supported by the fact that 'even after a delay of five years between suture and training, patients have improved considerably' (Wynn Parry, 1973).

Since Wynn Parry's pioneer work, systematic sensory retraining has been accepted as an integral part of the rehabilitation of patients after repair of the nerves supplying the hand. The subject has been greatly developed by Dellon (1988) who has both systematized the methods of sensory retraining and documented the results in a large number of patients. Dellon's studies are an invaluable source for anyone interested in the subject of sensory function.

Sensory re-education in Moscow

Another source of inspiration was a remarkable book by Leont'ev and Zaporozhets published in Moscow in 1945 and in English translation in 1960. 'Rehabilitation of the Hand' is a massive study of World War II patients with injuries of the upper limb. It describes the profound – one might say 'global' – disturbance of hand function in all its aspects wrought by these injuries, and the course and methods of restoration of function. Two themes are central to the book. The first is that 'a disturbance of a function of a limb cannot be explained by purely anatomical changes', the second that 'the restoration of damaged function by no means takes place by itself as an automatic consequence of regeneration of the tissues of the damaged organ'. Both themes imply a dissociation between anatomy and function in the severely wounded. These patients develop new modes of function – or dysfunction – not tightly linked to the anatomical injury, and they need more than anatomical repair in order to regain normal function.

Using simple but ingenious experimental apparatus with a large variety of patients, Leont'ev and Zaporozhets documented a remarkably uniform picture of discoordination, whether the patients had multiple fractures, contractures, amputations or nerve injuries. This led them to the view that 'the reorganization of the limb arising in connection with injury leads to its functional dissociation from the sensory–motor systems forming the higher mechanisms of motor behaviour' and that 'the central gnostic [i.e. cognitive] element of these systems, which first represented a particular organ, also appears dissociated'. Rehabilitation was therefore addressed first and foremost to restoring co-ordination of the injured limb – with the rest of the body and, more specifically, with the intact higher centres. Increase in strength and range of movement occurred only after improvement in co-ordination, and co-ordination was best acquired through the repetition of small 'functional' tasks containing a strong proprioceptive element and falling well within the limits of the patient's strength and range of movement.

From the point of view of sensory re-education, their most illuminating case studies are those of patients who underwent Krukenberg's operation after bilateral low amputation of the forearm. In this operation, after loss of the hand, the two bones of the forearm are separated surgically to form two new 'digits'. The use of these new digits was found to be ultimately dependent on their acquiring the sensory-perceptual function of the hand that they must replace. (Phillips [1986], discussing the Krukenberg arm, states that 'the threshold of two-point discrimination has been observed to improve from 16 mm, the normal value for forearm skin, to 8 to 10 mm'). Sensory re-education therefore played a crucial part in the patients' rehabilitation. This was done entirely through object recognition, the patient being led by questions to develop what the authors called 'tactics of perception'. For instance, a patient (blindfolded by goggles) is given a prism to palpate with his Krukenberg hand:

> **Subject:** This is something I don't know at all. It has angles. Has it got a name?
> **Experimenter:** Yes, every object here has a name.
> **Subject:** I don't think this has a name, but if... let me think now ... if there are many angles that means it may be called a polygon ... that's what we'll call it. Did I guess that or not? I am sure I must have made a mistake, this hand of mine feels very badly.

The authors describe this sort of partial faltering recognition as tactile agnosia, in which 'the hand satisfactorily distinguishes the shape and the individual elements of the object, but the patient is not aware of the object as a whole and he cannot say what it is'. At this stage, the movements of the digits have an arbitrary appearance, unrelated to the object which they are supposedly palpating. The first sign of developing object recognition (stereognosis) is the appearance of purposeful, systematic movements, or tactics of perception.

In another series of experiments, the authors examined the integration of sensory and visual information in their patients by means of the size–weight illusion known as the Charpentier test (Charpentier, 1891). This describes the common experience that, when two objects of equal weight are held in the hand and seen, the smaller of the two feels heavier – or a pound of lead feels heavier than a pound of feathers. Patients in the early period after the Krukenberg operation showed a reversed illusion, with judgement dictated purely by vision: a larger object, even if lighter, was pronounced heavier. This response is normally found only in young children (Yekutiel, Robin and Yarom, 1981). The appearance of a normal Charpentier illusion occurred before – and indeed predicted – the development of stereognosis. This evidence of the early integration of sensori-motor and visual information in the course of the recovery of sensory function provides a rationale for the central role of vision in Wynn Parry's method of sensory retraining described earlier (Wynn Parry, 1973).

Leont'ev and Zaporozhets looked beyond the traditional distinctions between musculoskeletal and nerve lesions and between the functions of the peripheral and central nervous systems and produced a study of patients and their recovery that has no rival.

In order to apply the lessons of these two studies of hand rehabilitation in peripheral injuries to the development of an approach to central sensory loss, it is useful to consider the causes of the sensory loss and the mechanisms of recovery in the peripheral cases and decide to what extent and in which way these are likely to differ in central cases.

Peripheral nerve lesions

The sensory disturbances in a patient during and after regeneration of a sutured nerve stem from a number of causes. However skilled the surgical technique of suture, repair can never be perfect. Some axons will fail altogether to cross the suture, and those that do cross are unlikely to grow into the exact endoneural tubes which they occupied formerly, or reach the end-organs which they innervated before (Sumner, 1990). Misalignment can be with a different type of end-organ (Koerber, Seymour and Mendell, 1989), with a similar end-organ in a different location (Horch, 1979), or a combination of both. In addition, nerve conduction velocity remains abnormally slow (Hallin, Wiesenfeld and Lindblom, 1981). Sensory input is therefore likely to be reduced, distorted and poorly localized (Dellon, 1988), and the patient needs to learn how to interpret and use it.

Another phenomenon which may add to the patient's confusion is the compensatory reaction of other nerves in the neighbourhood of the area formerly supplied by the severed nerve. Whether by sprouting into the denervated area or by activating pre-existing but unused branches, intact nerves near the area of sensory loss have been shown to provide some, albeit crude, substitution for the sensation lost (Weddell, Guttmann and Gutmann, 1941; Livingstone, 1947; Inbal et al., 1987; Healy, LeQuesne and Lynn, 1996). This can reduce the area of total anaesthesia and provide a measure of protective sensation. However, from the point of view of the long-term recovery of discriminative sensory function, this 'alien' afferent connection may be expected only to add to the confusion. If, as suggested by Inbal and colleagues, axons from the ulnar nerve can partially serve areas of skin denervated by a median nerve lesion, the messages which these axons convey to the brain will carry false or at best unclear information about their place of origin. When the regenerating median nerve reinervates the periphery, there seems to be some process of withdrawal or inhibition which reduces the activity of the ulnar substitution (Devor et al.,

1979), but it is not known when or to what degree this occurs or to what extent the regenerated median nerve regains its former dominance in the peripheral afferent field.

In addition to the effects of misalignment of regenerating nerve fibres and of possible confusion due to invasion by intact nerves, there is a third cause of poor function after peripheral nerve lesion. Before the introduction of sensory retraining, few patients regained more than crude protective sensation after suture and regeneration of the median nerve (Wynn Parry, 1973). Even if motor function recovered well, the hand was clumsy and patients learned to avoid using it, for instance by keeping their money in the other pocket. This will recall the phenomenon of 'learned non-use' described in Chapter 3. It undoubtedly exacerbated the poor sensory recovery of these early patients.

Central effects

This brings us to consider what happens in the brain when a peripheral nerve is cut. Recall that a peripheral nerve, such as the median nerve which innervates most of the palmar side of the hand and fingers, transmits its sensory information to the contralateral cerebral cortex via a series of relay stations in the spinal cord and brain which are linked by nerve tracts. Although nerves from all over the skin and deeper tissues converge upon this route, they are arranged in an orderly fashion at every station on the way, and their topographical origin and the modality or type of message that they carry are preserved throughout. Their main destination, after the last relay in the thalamic nuclei and the projection through the internal capsule, is the somatosensory cortex. Here they terminate in a map – actually, a set of maps (Kaas et al., 1979) – of the body extending laterally from the receptive area for the toes close to the midline of the brain, via areas for the leg, trunk, neck, shoulder and arm, to the area for the hand and fingers on the lateral aspect of the cerebral hemisphere, just above the area for the face. This map, often known as the 'homunculus', is a rather distorted image of the body since the area devoted to each body part bears little relation to the part's actual size but is instead proportional to its importance in sensory perception. Each finger (and each lip) gets a larger area than the whole leg or trunk (Penfield and Boldrey, 1937), and the thumb and index finger have larger representations than the other fingers (Sutherling, Levesque and Baumgartner, 1992). The sensory input is arranged in similar maps in the afferent (incoming) columns of the spinal cord and in the thalamic nuclei.

It has been known for over two decades that loss of peripheral input is followed by changes in the organization of the sensory cortex. This is so whether the peripheral input is removed by section of a peripheral nerve, by amputation of a digit or other organ, or by section of the dorsal (sensory) roots of peripheral nerves in the spinal cord. It might be expected that after complete removal of peripheral input the receptive area in the sensory cortex would be for ever 'silent', that it would not be possible to produce an evoked potential by any stimulus. However, this is not so. After a variable period of silence, the deprived cortex begins to respond to stimulation of skin adjacent to the amputated digit or denervated skin area, and a gradual reorganization occurs in the sensory cortex. This has been repeatedly documented in animals, especially in those like raccoons and monkeys which have highly developed tactile and manipulative abilities and correspondingly enlarged and well defined cortical representation of the hands. In Rasmusson's classic study of the cortical effects of amputating the fifth finger in adult raccoons, the cortical receptive field for this finger had been taken over almost entirely by input from the fourth finger by 16 weeks (Rasmusson, 1982). Similar effects are produced by section of a peripheral nerve. Merzenich and Kaas, working with monkeys, cut the median nerve which innervates some 60% of the palmar side of the hand and found the cortical receptive area gradually taken over by input from the adjoining ulnar-innervated area of the hand and the radial-innervated back of the hand (Merzenich and Kaas, 1982). The detailed topographical organization of these 'new' receptive fields varies greatly between different areas, between different animals and within the same animal at different periods of post-operative time. It is in general less orderly than the pre-operative organization (Wall et al., 1986). From these and other studies, it is clear that the same cortical area can come to represent different peripheral areas, depending on what part of the peripheral input is lost (Kaas, 1991).

These are only two examples from a large body of experimental work (Merzenich and Jenkins, 1993), all attesting to what Katz (1993) has called 'the cortical space race', or the competition between afferent inputs for connections in the sensory cortex. If the normal input is cut off, another input takes over. This neuroplasticity is not limited to the cortex, but occurs at every level of the central nervous system, including possibly the other cerebral hemisphere (Calford and Tweedale, 1990). Microelectrodes implanted in the cortex and subcortical relay stations on the sensory path between the face and the cortex in rats showed new responses to other facial areas within minutes of the deactivation of their usual sensory input (Faggin, Nguyen and Nicolelis, 1997). Functional reorganization after deafferentation has also been demonstrated in the dorsal horn cells of the spinal cord (Koerber and Mirnics, 1996) and in the thalamus (Garraghty and Kaas, 1991; Rasmusson, 1996).

From the point of view of a patient recovering from a peripheral nerve lesion we see that parallel with the peripheral changes in sensory input brought about by the gradual regeneration of the sutured nerve, as well as by possible compensatory responses in neighbouring nerves, the receptive fields in the central nervous system are also changing. There is thus a dynamic process of reorganization going forward at every level from the periphery up to the cortex, and recovery of function cannot be understood without considering the role of central factors (Braune and Schady, 1993). Little is known about what happens in the domains of perception beyond the primary sensory cortex, but Oliver Sack's enthralling account of 'the cerebral resonances' of his own peripheral injury (Sacks, 1984) provides much food for thought.

The effects of behaviour

To what extent is neural reorganization influenced by the behaviour of the patient? Does the changing cortical map react to his or her using or not using the affected hand? If the improvement in sensory function during retraining comes through learning to interpret abnormal sensations, what is the neurophysiological basis of this learning? Would it be possible with micro-electrodes to find some visible reflection of the patient's progress in the form of an increasingly extensive, orderly and discrete sensory map in the cortex?

Research using sophisticated techniques for imaging the activity of the brain during various kinds of behaviour has brought us to the threshold of being able to answer these questions, but the evidence – some from animals, some from humans – is still indirect and the application to the rehabilitation of neurological patients still tentative. The animal studies will be reviewed first.

Healthy adult monkeys were taught that the only way to get food was by keeping their second and third finger tips lightly in contact with the edge of a rotating disc. They did this for up to two hours a day for several weeks. Mapping of the finger area in the somatosensory cortex before and after this period showed a large expansion – threefold in some cases – of the area for these two finger tips (Jenkins et al., 1990). This study was followed by a series of experiments in which monkeys learned to discriminate progressively smaller differences in the frequency of vibratory tactile stimulation applied to a constant point on a digit (Recanzone, Merzenich and Jenkins, 1992a). The sensory cortical area representing this point showed progressive enlargement, both compared with areas not stimulated and compared with monkeys who received the same vibratory stimulation while attending to an auditory task. This led the authors to conclude that 'stimulation alone is far less efficient in driving cortical reorganization when compared with actively discriminating the stimulus'. Changes induced by training were found not only in the cortical area 3b, considered the main area involved in tactile discrimination, but also in the adjacent area 3a whose dominant input is from muscle stretch receptors, suggesting that these neurons may be recruited when needed in a cutaneous task (Recanzone et al., 1992b). These are just a few of the findings supporting the conclusion that 'remodeling of the details of cortical representations parallels the development or improvement of new skills and behaviors throughout life, and plausibly accounts for them' (Recanzone, Merzenich and Shreiner, 1992c). The cortical changes were brought about, not by simple stimulation of the monkey's hand, but by involving the animal's attention in discriminating the sensory stimuli for the sake of a reward. Another study recorded the changes in sensory cortical activity as monkeys switched their attention from a visual detection task to a tactile discriminatory one (Hsiao, O'Shaughnessy and Johnson, 1993).

Although other research has confirmed this remodeling of the sensory cortex after enhanced use in various experimental procedures in animals, there is always a slight doubt about extrapolating animal findings to man. However, an elegant study of the sensory cortex in 15 blind subjects who habitually read Braille with the right index finger showed significant expansion of the cortical representation of this finger compared with the left non-reading index finger or with index fingers of control subjects (Pascual-Leone and Torres, 1993). Braille is read by making small side-to-side scanning movements of the reading index finger, and the motor cortical area targeting one of the muscles used in this movement was found to be significantly larger than that related to a lateral mover of another finger (Pascual-Leone et al., 1993). An even more dramatic reorganization of brain function in habitual Braille readers is the activation of the visual cortex not only during Braille reading but also during the performance of non-Braille tactile discriminatory tasks (Sadato et al., 1996).

Pascual-Leone and his colleagues have also recorded changes in the spatial extension and intensity of motor cortical output to hand muscles during different types of manual skill acquisition. In perhaps their most interesting study (Pascual-Leone et al., 1995), transcranial magnetic stimulation was used to map the area of the motor cortex targeting the long flexor and extensor muscles of the hand over a period of five days while subjects did either physical or mental practice of a 5-finger piano exercise for two hours a day. Performance improved in both groups, though significantly more with physical practice than with mental practice. The most striking finding was that both physical and mental practice was accompanied by a large increase in the number of scalp sites from which the finger muscles could be excited, implying an increase in the size of the cortical representation of the muscles involved. There was also a decrease in their threshold of activation. These findings concern predominantly motor areas of the cortex. Another 'musical' study focusing on the sensory cortex of people who have played the violin or other string instruments for many years found a marked enlargement of the sensory cortical representation of the fingers of their left hands (Elbert et al., 1995).

These studies indicate that the distribution and size of the cortical representation of the fingers are influenced by learning and by active use, and this has been shown in humans as well as in experimental animals.

How does a cortical neuron, which regularly responded to input from one finger, change to responding to a different finger? Twenty-five years ago, when the early experiments in this field were carried out, the adult brain was still considered to be 'hard-wired', with its pathways laid down *in utero* or in early childhood. Much discussion was devoted to whether the cortical reorganization should be attributed to anatomical changes, such as axonal growth, sprouting and the formation of new synapses, or to functional changes such as the unmasking – by activation or by disinhibition – of existing but hitherto non-functioning connections. Although the controversy has not been finally resolved (Stroemer, Kent and Hulsebosch, 1995; Elliott, Howarth and Shadbolt, 1996), there has been a major change in the perception of the nature of the brain, away from the rigid conceptions of classical neurology and towards the recognition that 'knowing a neuron's name and address doesn't assure knowledge of its function' (Klopfer, 1992). Study of the micro-structure of the brain has revealed a multiplicity of intraneural connections such as 'would allow each cortical neuron, which undoubtedly receives many different kinds of inputs and projects to various targets, to be selected for, and thus to participate in, simultaneously, more than one kind of functional unit' (White, 1989). At the same time, research is elucidating the role of excitatory and inhibitory neurotransmitters in determining the relative strength of the synapses on individual neurons. This subject takes us beyond the scope of this book, but it is encouraging to note that it is already possible to build a tentative model of the neuro-chemical processes underlying the cortical reorganization which takes place both in response to the loss of sensory input and during acquisition of a new skill (Dykes, 1997; Fazeli and Collingridge, 1997).

Central lesions

We come now to consider sensory disturbance caused not by a loss of input from the periphery but by damage to the brain itself. After small focal lesions in the hand area of monkeys' somatosensory cortex, there is extensive reorganization of the surrounding cortex by which 'most of the skin surface formerly represented in a small infarcted zone comes to be represented topographically in the cortical region around it, with both the original representations in this area and the new ones occupying slightly smaller areas than before' (Jenkins and Merzenich, 1987). This is encouraging, but we must repeat the caveat about applying findings from monkey to man. Sixty years ago, Ruch, Fulton and German showed that the sensory loss caused by anatomically comparable parietal lesions becomes more severe and less reversible as one passes from monkey to chimpanzee and from chimpanzee to man, indicating a progressive corticalization of somatic sensation (Ruch, Fulton and German, 1938). The main importance of their paper, however, lies in its being perhaps the earliest mention of the possibility of sensory retraining after brain damage. Chimpanzees, trained to get their food by discriminating weights, textures or geometrical shapes, developed varying deficits in these abilities after each of a series of parietal ablations but recovered most – sometimes all – discriminative ability after retraining. The retraining was not started until several weeks after the operation in order to separate its effects from those of postoperative recovery. 'The efficacy of retraining in promoting recovery is shown by an analysis of daily scores, which demonstrates that great improvement may occur within a training series, between consecutive days and even within the daily training session.' Four patients with surgical parietal lesions showed greater deficits and less recovery, but 'it is possible that comparable amounts of retraining would further reduce the postoperative incapacity in man'. Strange and disappointing that the authors did not think to give their human patients the benefit of the sensory retraining so effective in their animal patients!

The last few years have seen the development of non-invasive techniques, such as positron emission tomography (PET) and magnetic resonance imaging (MRI), which have made it possible to study the damaged human brain during recovery. These methods provide a fascinating picture of the different routes by which the brain can recuperate lost or disordered functions.

A group at the Hammersmith Hospital in London used PET scanning of regional blood-flow to study brain function in patients after recovery from stroke (Chollett et al., 1991; Weiller et al., 1992; Weiller et al, 1993). Scanning of patients while they used their previously paralyzed hands to perform thumb opposition to each finger in turn – an operation normally accompanied by activity in the contralateral hemisphere – showed unusual activity in the ipsilateral (unaffected) motor cortex and parietal cortex and in the cerebellum. In addition to this apparent recruitment of brain areas far from the usual focus of activity during this task, the area of focal activity was larger than normal, indicating an apparent extension of the 'motor map' (Chollett and Weiller, 1994). Although all the patients were considered to have made a complete recovery, there were considerable individual differences in their patterns of brain activity during finger opposition, presumably related to the site and extent of the stroke.

Cerebral activity has also been studied during a tactile discrimination task in stroke patients whose motor function had recovered after complete initial loss of hand function (Weder et al., 1994). As well as activation of sensory and motor cortical hand areas ipsilateral to the lesion, there were differences between patients which could be related both to the site of lesion and to the patients' performance on the sensory tests. Other similar studies have also found evidence of ipsilateral involvement in the motor recovery of stroke patients (Caramia, Iani and Bernardi, 1996; Silvestrini et al., 1993). There are also indications that the right hemisphere may be involved in recovery from aphasia after stroke (Thomas et al., 1997).

Years before this documentation of the role of the contralateral hemisphere in recovery after unilateral brain lesions, there were reports of remarkable recovery in patients after the surgical removal of one hemisphere (Griffith and Davidson, 1966; Glees, 1986). These operations were carried out mostly in children, but also in young adults, for the relief of intractable epilepsy. Glees, for instance, described two patients – one whose left hemisphere was removed at the age of 20, the other his right hemisphere at 19 – who made good recoveries, showing that 'one hemisphere is sufficient to sustain a personality in locomotion, sensory perception of the whole body, speech and in relatively normal social contact with his environment'. More recently, modern methods of mapping brain function have shown reorganized cortical representation of ipsilateral muscles alongside the usual areas for contralateral muscles in the remaining hemisphere in patients like these (Benecke, Meyer and Fruend, 1991; Cohen et al., 1993).

Another piece of evidence for the role of the intact hemisphere in recovery comes from reports of patients making a good functional recovery after unilateral stroke only to be paralyzed again – this time on both sides – by a second stroke in the opposite hemisphere. Fisher (1992) reported two such cases, both patients with pure motor stroke affecting the left side, who were regaining voluntary movement when a second stroke on the opposite side robbed them of the use of both the right side of the body and of the returning movement of the left side. A similar case was recently reported by Lee and van Donkelaar (1995).

In spite of the weight of these different lines of evidence, the role of the undamaged hemisphere in recovery of function is still controversial. It should be noted that a number of studies found no evidence for ipsilateral involvement in the recovery of patients' control of muscles previously paralysed by stroke (Palmer, Ashby and Hajek 1992; Traversa et al., 1997; Bastings et al., 1997). It seems likely that the contradictory findings may reflect, on the one hand, differences in the procedures used – both the techniques of measurement and the demands on the patient – and, on the other hand, different patterns of brain reorganization in response to injury.

From the studies reviewed, there emerge the following general conclusions about cerebral activity in recovered stroke patients: 1) brain areas remote from the site of damage are recruited, including in many cases the intact hemisphere; 2) sites adjacent to the lesion may show unusual activity during performance of a task normally involving the damaged area; and 3) the pattern of cerebral activity varies greatly between patients and can be related on the one hand to the site and extent of the stroke and on the other hand to the degree of recovery. Stroke is followed by functional cerebral reorganization involving many regions and both sides of the brain, and the marked individual differences observed show that various possibilities exist for cerebral reorganization and the recovery of function.

The clear link between cerebral reorganization after stroke and the patient's recuperation of lost abilities poses again the question raised in the review of neuroplasticity in peripheral lesions: namely, to what extent is the process of recovery – cerebral and behavioural – influenced by what the patient does, by his or her environment or by any form of therapy?

In the absence of answers from human studies, we have to fall back on animal studies. There is a large volume of literature beginning in the 1960s on the effects of enriched environment on brain size and structure in both developing and adult rodents (Rosenzweig, Bennett and Diamond 1972; Walsh, 1981; Rosenzweig and Bennett, 1996), and these studies have recently been extended to rats subjected to a typical stroke by surgical ligature of one middle cerebral artery (Ohlsson and Johansson, 1995; B.B. Johansson, 1996). Rats kept after the operation in an enriched environment – in a large cage with other rats and with a variety of swings, climbing blocks and other challenging objects – showed greater recovery of locomotor abilities (balancing, climbing, and the like) than those kept alone in individual standard cages. Even better results were obtained when the animals were kept in the enriched environment for eight pre-operative weeks as well as in the post-operative period.

Mountcastle (1975), monitoring activity in the parietal cortex of monkeys, observed that 'neurons discharge at much higher rates during active movements emitted by the animal than during passive ones imposed by the experimenter', and the importance of the animal's attention and motivation has been demonstrated in plasticity-inducing conditioning experiments (Ahissar et al., 1992), as well as in the studies of Recanzone and colleagues (1992a–c) and Hsiao, O'Shaughnessy and Johnson (1993) described above. The response of cortical cells tends to decline with repeated stimulation (Condon and Weinberger, 1991), and it seems likely that the thresholds of cortical neurons for potentiation or depression are not fixed, but rather controlled or at least influenced by some 'gating' mechanism related to behaviourally relevant factors (Cruikshank and Weinberger, 1996).

Nudo and colleagues, studying the motor cortical hand map in monkeys before and after subjecting them to small ischaemic infarcts at identified regions of this map, found that the ensuing changes in cortical function were markedly influenced by whether the animals were given 'rehabilitative training' (Nudo et al., 1996). Monkeys who had learned to use their fingers to get food pellets out of small wells lost this skill after the infarct, but recovered their original levels of performance after 3–4 weeks of what the authors describe as 'an intensive behavioral retraining procedure'. Motor cortical maps in monkeys not given this retraining showed no new representation of the functional area lost, but instead a further loss of hand territory in the area surrounding the infarct. In the rehabilitated monkeys, however, this further loss did not occur; there was instead a significant expansion of the undamaged hand and wrist area into areas formerly serving the elbow and shoulder.

Guidelines for intervention

In 1986, Phillips ended his Sherrington lectures on movements of the hand with the statement that 'the plasticity of somaesthetic and motor maps will have to be understood before it can be controlled for the benefit of patients' (Phillips, 1986). Since then the study of neuroplasticity has flourished, and the time has come to use the new insights for the benefit of patients.

What have we learned from the search for a rational basis for the rehabilitation of sensory function after stroke? Two key statements can be made. First, the possibility of sensory recovery rests entirely in the functional plasticity of the brain. Second, the functional organization of the brain is use-dependent, and neuroplasticity is an adaptive response to demand.

Certain themes recur throughout the studies on the reorganization of neural function in animals and man. It is worth highlighting these themes and considering their relevance to therapy for stroke patients with sensory loss.

The brain responds to meaningful demands

Functional cerebral reorganization after injury (peripheral or central) can take many forms, and the form it takes is profoundly influenced by the demands made on the nervous system. This is another way of saying that it is adaptive to the needs of the organism. From the material reviewed in this chapter, it is clear that meaningful tasks – as opposed to meaningless stimuli – are necessary for functional neuroplasticity. The crucial role of motivated behaviour in driving cortical reorganization is a central finding of many of the studies reviewed. The work of Nudo and his colleagues shows that neural reorganization after damage to the sensory cortex can range from beneficial to detrimental (Nudo et al., 1996). If no special demands are made, as in the unrehabilitated monkeys, dysfunction may spread to cortical areas adjacent to the infarct, whereas if the monkeys have to depend on their hands to get their food – and are trained intensively in this skill – cortical reorganization provides a larger hand area, even at the expense of more proximal limb areas not essential to the skill.

These studies highlight the importance of the goal of behaviour and its paramount influence on function, in sickness and in health. Although we are all familiar with the fact that when a dog hurts its leg it immediately changes to walking on three legs, and our own daily lives are replete with automatic adaptations of behaviour which allow us to pursue our goals despite bodily or environmental constraints, an ecological understanding of the behaviour of patients has been long in coming. It may be natural for a biologist to interpret an organism's response to disease or trauma as adaptively geared to its functioning and survival, but it is only recently that this way of thinking has begun to infiltrate the mindset of people concerned with disability and rehabilitation. Largely due to the work of non-medical researchers, abnormal gait and other 'clinical signs' of pathology are beginning to be interpreted as optimal solutions to the problems posed to the patient by that pathology (Marshall and Jennings, 1990; Mulder, 1991). It has even been suggested that spasticity may promote – rather than hinder – function in the brain-damaged (Burke, 1988). The behaviour of a hemiplegic patient, who uses only one hand and walks with a stiff and asymmetrical gait, does indeed present the typical clinical picture of a unilateral cerebral lesion. But this behaviour can also be recognized as the brain's way of meeting the patient's demands in spite of the restrictions imposed by the pathology. This euphoric view should perhaps be tempered by noting that although the compensatory strategies produced by the brain represent optimal solutions for achieving immediate goals, their influence can sometimes be deleterious in the long run (LeVere and LeVere, 1982; Shepherd and Carr, 1991). In spite of this reservation, one can only welcome the infusion of biological concepts into the approach to disability. The mental switch to an ecological or dynamical systems approach – with its emphasis on the goals of behaviour – has profound implications for rehabilitation therapy which have only begun to be explored by therapists (Shepherd and Carr, 1991). In the next chapter, we shall see that there are signs of a similar influence of biological thinking in the area of mental and emotional problems after stroke.

Damage to an animal's brain seems to put into high gear the processes of functional reorganization which have been going on throughout its life. Luria (1963) wrote: 'An essential condition of such a reorganization [of function] is that the particular activity is needed by the animal, and the greater the need the more easily and automatically will the required reorganization take place'. The challenge is now greater, the constraints more serious, but the overall goal is still to function and to survive. Whether the sensory systems have been affected or remain intact, the brain damage must have increased the amount of what Gregory (1961) – in an analogy to the static in radio communication – called 'the neural noise levels' in the brain and thus heightened the risk of confusion between signals. The last thing that the beleaguered brain needs is any addition to the level of 'noise' in the nervous system: indeed, one of its immediate tasks must be to minimize noise. Meaningless stimulation, by increasing the ratio of noise to information, can only add to the brain's problem of concentrating its remaining forces on the perceptions and actions that matter.

The application of animal studies to man

Can we apply the results of studies of rats, cats and monkeys to man? Perhaps, along with other traits, we have lost some of the great neuroplasticity found in other mammals. Such a possibility is in the first place intuitively implausible: without our enormous capacity to learn we would surely not have survived as a species. But the argument need not rely only on intuition. Two lines of evidence attest to the human brain's remarkable capacity for functional reorganization in response to experience. The first comes from the studies of Pascual-Leone and his colleagues. People learning skilled finger movements show the same sort of changes in cortical activity seen in monkeys trained to use their fingers for a reward

(Pascual-Leone et al., 1995). Habitual Braille readers, blind from early childhood, not only have an enlarged sensory cortical area for their Braille reading finger but also appear to use their visual cortex in other – non-reading – tasks of tactile discrimination (Pascual-Leone and Torres, 1993; Sadato et al., 1996).

The other line of evidence for neuroplasticity in man as well as in animals comes from studies of brain activity in people who have recovered from stroke. When the damage to the brain is permanent, recovery of function can be mediated only by functional reorganization of the remaining intact areas. A great variety of reorganized patterns of cerebral activity has been observed, including heightened activity in the neighbourhood of the lesion, in other areas on the same side of the brain and in the undamaged side of the brain. The reorganization of function within the brain seems to vary from patient to patient. The primary factor determining what pattern of reorganization occurs must presumably be the nature of the lesion – its rate of development, site and extent and its repercussions throughout the brain. But, in the light of our review of neuroplasticity, the brain's response to the injury must also be influenced by the lifetime experience of the patient and his or her brain – not only by what he or she experienced before the stroke, but overwhelmingly by experiences after the stroke.

Lesions of the peripheral nerves and lesions within the central nervous system

When a peripheral nerve is cut, the brain's link with that area of the body – its skin, muscles and joints – is lost. Until the nerve is sutured and the slow process of regeneration well under way, all that the brain can do is to 'lease' the deprived central areas to some other input. When the nerve finally regenerates, neither the peripheral arrangement nor the cortical one is exactly as it was before the injury, and the outcome for the patient – especially as regards sensory function – is often less than satisfactory. Until sensory retraining was introduced for these patients, their treatment consisted of intensive exercise to activate and strengthen paralysed muscles, and the use of splints, passive stretching and massage to prevent contracture and to maintain and increase range of joint movement. For motor function, the results of this treatment were often good, but – in the case of the nerves supplying the hand – sensory recovery was poor: most patients recovered little more than protective sensation, and without sensory discrimination the hand was clumsy. The poor sensory recovery was not due to lack of stimulation, since the regime of massage and passive stretching was vigorous and often painful. But such stimuli, given to a passive patient, bear no resemblance to the type of meaningful challenges found to drive cortical reorganization. By contrast, the sensory retraining developed by Wynn Parry posed interesting and varied puzzles to the recovering sensory system, and 70 per cent of his patients with median nerve lesions regained good sensory function (Wynn Parry, 1973). In the light of research reviewed from the last twenty years, it is logical to suppose that these patients learned to interpret and use unfamiliar sensory input and that this learning was mediated by cerebral reorganization.

In the case of stroke, the damage is to the much more plastic central nervous system. The irreplaceable peripheral nervous system remains intact and continues to transmit faithfully to the central nervous system. The clinical picture of sensory loss after stroke, as we saw in Chapter 3, is almost never the total and sharply localized anaesthesia that occurs when a peripheral nerve is cut. The greater plasticity of the central nervous system stems from its multiplicity of pathways. While the sensory information from, say, the tip of the index finger has one sole path of access to the central nervous system (namely, the median nerve), and it is relayed fully and exactly to the contralateral sensory cortex, it passes through stations on the way – notably in the thalamus – which connect directly and indirectly with many other brain areas. Sensory information is, for instance, passed directly from the thalamus to the motor cortex as well as via the somatosensory cortex. There are also relays to the ipsilateral side of the brain at all levels: by uncrossed paths, by paths which cross and recross, as well as through the various commissures connecting the two halves of the brain. It is indeed not surprising that the picture of functional cerebral reorganization is so varied in stroke patients who have regained the use of their hands.

If, without sensory retraining, peripheral nerve patients find their hands clumsy and get used to not using them even if their motor function has recovered, this tendency to 'learned non-use' must be a major factor in the behaviour of a stroke patient with sensory loss. In addition to whatever motor and other impairments the stroke has caused, the residue of sensory information that does 'get through' may be so reduced and so distorted as to be of little immediate use to the brain. This 'noise' is likely to activate processes of descending inhibition which, even if not compounded by central neglect, will foster learned non-use. The detrimental effect of learned non-use on recovery after stroke can be inferred from the very positive functional effects of a programme of 'forced use' in which stroke patients were required to keep their 'good' hand and arm enclosed in a sling during waking hours (Wolf et al., 1989).

Sensory rehabilitation needs to be active, interesting and demanding

This, then, is the challenge: a patient with a sudden catastrophic insult to the brain, who has not only been struck by varying degrees of paralysis and cognitive impairment but also experiences a drastic loss of meaningful sensory connection with half the body.

The message from the neurophysiological literature is abundantly clear. The essential ingredients for any intervention which hopes to harness the brain's potential for functional reorganization and learning are: *motivation* and *attention*. Functional recovery of patients is likely to be fostered by the kind of experience provided by the 'enriched environment' found therapeutic in rats after cerebral infarction (Ohlsson and Johansson, 1995; B.B. Johansson, 1996): namely, intense occupation in interesting and varied activities in a socially stimulating, rather than an isolated situation.

Unfortunately, the daily life of patients hospitalized after stroke presents a picture far removed from the enriched environment given to these rodents! Out of a potential 8-hour day for rehabilitation, patients spend over 60% of the time alone and a bare 3.4% to 7.5% in therapy (Wade et al., 1984; Lincoln et al., 1996). Although the situation is slightly better in rehabilitation settings than in general hospitals, 'in all settings observed, patients spent many hours sitting and doing nothing' (Lincoln et al. 1996). It should be noted that the latter paper was written *after* an attempt had been made to remedy the situation (Tinson, 1989). By contrast, in Chessington and Moscow – the two centres which pioneered the idea of sensory retraining – the patients were kept busy with their rehabilitation for the whole of the working day (Wynn Parry, 1973; Leont'ev and Zaporozhets, 1945/1960). As regards the quality of therapy, the emphasis in both places was on meaningful and motivating activity. In both situations it was, of course, a matter of rehabilitating young servicemen and either returning them to work or paying disability compensation. Even if such *intensity* of therapy cannot be achieved in civilian settings and with older patients, much can be learned from these studies about the *quality* of therapy required for sensory rehabilitation. A style of therapy is needed which poses interesting and meaningful challenges to the brain, is designed to avoid monotony at all costs and alert attention – in short, to recruit the brain's enormous capacity for functional reorganization. The patient is not a machine left by the driver to be serviced: it is the driver who needs help, and the passive role allotted to the patient in so much of current therapy is more likely to depress cortical activity than to foster it.

Chapter 5
Contributions from psychology

The previous chapter concluded that sensory rehabilitation needs to be active, interesting and demanding if it is to harness the brain's great potential for adaptive functional reorganization. In monkeys, learning and reorganization of brain function can be achieved by the simple procedure of offering a reward of juice or banana pellets for mastering a new task, or even by making this behaviour the animals' only way to get food. In humans the situation is not so simple, and in stroke patients it is vastly more complex. We clearly need help from the psychologists.

Therapists – notably physiotherapists, but also occupational therapists – are trained and experienced in dealing with predominantly 'physical' problems. As regards 'psychological' problems, they are expected to be aware of them, even on the lookout for them, but not to treat them. For many physiotherapists this area is, in fact, almost taboo, (which may explain – though not justify – the meagre contribution made by physiotherapy in the areas of health education, preventive medicine and mental health). For sensory re-education after stroke, this professional barrier has to be broached. The neurophysiologists have linked up with the psychologists in the study of the brain, and the physiotherapists need to make a similar alliance in order to enrich their agenda for the brain-damaged patient. Although little has been written about teaching and learning with direct reference to stroke patients, there is a large psychological literature to be culled for relevant insights. The following very eclectic review is arranged around the subjects of attention and motivation and their bearing on learning.

Attention

'Everyone knows what attention is', wrote William James and proceeded to define it as:

the taking possession of the mind, in clear and vivid form, of one out of what seem several simultaneously possible objects or trains of thought. Focalization, concentration, of consciousness are of its essence. It implies withdrawal from some things in order to deal effectively with others, and is a condition which has a real opposite in the confused, dazed, scatter-brained state.... called distraction (James, 1890).

James uses the term to describe both a cause and an effect: a spotlight to be focused when one pays attention and a resulting state of 'focalization, concentration of consciousness', and the quotation from James already shows that, even if everyone knows what attention is, it is surely a complex phenomenon with many components. Posner, for instance, defined three 'senses of attention' (Posner and Boies, 1971; Posner and Rafal, 1987). These are: general alertness or arousal (which can refer to tonic or phasic attention), selective attention, and sustained concentration or vigilance.

The study of attention

Along with many other attributes of the mind, attention was an unacceptable subject for study during the reign of behaviorist psychology, but it came to occupy a central position in the rapid rise of cognitive psychology from the 1960s onwards (Eysenck and Keane, 1990). Though clearly a feature of all sensory-perceptual systems – for one can attend to a smell, a sound, a sight or a touch, as well as to a thought or a memory – it was first studied in the auditory sphere, for instance in the 'cocktail party phenomenon' or the process of attending to one voice out of a barrage of noise (Cherry, 1957). Research then moved on to vision, and visual attention has since dominated the field. Under the combined influence of the long tradition of localization of brain functions and the contemporary development of information theory and computers, there was a vigorous search for a simple unitary theory of attention and for an anatomical site for the control of attention. Various sorts of 'filter' were postulated to select between incoming stimuli, one of the earliest being that proposed by Broadbent (1958) which filtered input into a 'limited-capacity system' at an early stage in processing on the basis of purely physical stimulus characteristics. In a move away from the information-processing models of attention, Neisser (1967) stressed the active conscious choice of information involved in attention, and filters were postulated at a later stage of processing and based on the behavioural relevance of the stimuli (Deutsch and Deutsch, 1963), or at variable stages and with flexible amounts of filtering (Treisman, 1969). On the localization issue, a major role in the control of directed attention was assigned to the right cerebral hemisphere (Brain, 1941), more particularly its parietal lobe (Denny-Brown and Chambers, 1958). However, the fact that patients can develop various types of unilateral neglect after lesions in a number of other areas suggested that 'the direction of attention towards sensory events within the extrapersonal space is modulated by a complex network which contains not only subcortical but also extensive cortical components' (Mesulam, 1981). For visual attention, two different systems have long been distinguished – functionally and anatomically – depending on whether the task involves simply identifying something ('what?') or locating it ('where?'). The former, object-identification system is identified with a ventral path from the visual cortex to the inferior temporal cortex, while the 'where' or visual location system runs more dorsally to the posterior parietal cortex (Ungerlieder and Mishkin, 1982). The 'where' system has more recently been conceived as mediating visual perception geared to action (Goodale and Milner, 1992). Visual attention thus has more than one neural substrate, and the attentional systems of other less studied senses are likely to be at least as multifaceted. As with the related subject of neglect, it is now clear that 'attentional functions are of many different kinds, serving a great range of different computational purposes. There can be no simple theory of attention, any more than there can be a simple theory of thought' (Allport,1993).

A stroke may damage this set of 'attentional functions' in many different ways, and this damage occurs for the most part in brains that have passed their age of optimal function.

The effects of ageing and the effects of stroke

Ageing brings with it a decline in many aspects of attention. Elderly people are more easily distracted by irrelevant information (Rabbitt, 1965), are less able to retrieve previously learned material (Haaland et al., 1987) and poor at maintaining sustained attention (Chao and Knight, 1997), and many of these deficits can be linked to prefrontal cortical and subcortical changes found in pathological and neurophysiological studies of the brain in elderly subjects (Chao and Knight, 1997). This is the main age group that suffers stroke, and it is important to remember that this catastrophe hits people who are to varying degrees already handicapped by declining powers of attention, concentration and memory. Stroke itself has a deleterious effect on cognitive functions, among them attention (Tatemichi et al., 1994; Kase et al., 1998). Many stroke patients are undoubtedly in 'the confused, dazed, scatter-brained state' which James described as the opposite of attention and labelled 'distraction' (James, 1890). Confusion, disorientation, inattention and various degrees of neglect and denial are found in a high proportion of patients in the first weeks after stroke (Marshall et al., 1997), often without a clear relation to the site of the primary damage. As time passes, much of this general disturbance of cognitive function resolves. The persistence of neglect, denial or other signs of disturbed awareness carries a very poor prognosis for recovery of function and forms one of what Adams and Hurwitz called the 'mental barriers to recovery' which they found characterized a 'hard-core of chronic hemiplegic invalids' (Adams and Hurwitz, 1963). Persistent neglect is commoner in right than in left hemisphere stroke, but it is important to note that it is far from rare in left hemisphere stroke: three months after stroke, 33% of left and 75% of right hemisphere stroke patients showed neglect (Stone et al., 1991). Even these figures probably underestimate the frequency and persistence of attentional problems in patients recovering from stroke. The prevalence of attentional problems in left hemisphere stroke is likely to be underestimated because their existence is difficult to determine in aphasic patients. More generally, testing of stroke patients for attention and neglect is commonly limited to visual tasks with static stimuli and to the performance of one task at a time. It is possible to do well on this sort of laboratory test but to have troublesome problems of inattention in the multidimensional situations of everyday life. Dittmar and Gliner (1987) found significant deficit in stroke patients' performance when they had to attend alternately to a visual and an acoustic task. This sort of switching or sharing of one's attention between listening and looking is a common feature of everyday life; it is also a basic requirement of a stroke patient trying to carry out a therapist's instructions. Marshall and colleagues compared patients living in the community between one and ten years after stroke with age-matched controls on a dynamic dual visual task involving tracking one moving target and detecting another which appeared intermittently. None of the subjects showed any signs of neglect on standard tests, and the patients performed as well as the controls on the continuous tracking task, whether performed as a single test or as part of a dual task. But both left and right hemisphere stroke patients performed less well than controls on target identification when this was combined with tracking, suggesting that 'individuals with prior stroke have less of an ability to divide their attention for competing tasks' (Marshall et al., 1997).

Sensory Re-education (SRE) clearly has to be geared to patients who are potentially distractible and likely to find it hard to concentrate and to sustain attention. This dictates certain basic requirements for SRE which will be considered now. As we leave the realm of statistics and approach the patient and therapist embarking on SRE, our task will be made easier if, for the sake of clarity, we choose as protagonists a male patient ('he') and a female therapist ('she').

Interest

The most important requirement for Sensory Re-education is that the patient should find the work interesting and thus rewarding for its own sake. Much of what is demanded of the patient in rehabilitation can be done without a great deal of mental effort, but SRE needs his full attention. 'Learning takes place as the result of active mental processing' (Howe, 1998), and SRE must therefore be sufficiently interesting to engage his attention. What does this mean? If we turn to 'interesting' in Webster's dictionary, we find: 'engaging the attention, capable of arousing interest, curiosity, or emotion'; and for synonyms: 'engrossing, absorbing, intriguing'. Further on, we have: 'Interesting may imply a power to provoke attentive interest ... through some such quality as curiosity, sympathy, desire to understand, enthusiasm ...' (Webster, 1966). These definitions highlight the *active* aspect of interest, the curiosity that leads to the exploration of something intriguing. This quality of active exploration is the essence of sensory-perceptual function, expressed so well by Peter Nathan:

> Philosophers and many psychologists used to believe that animals, including ourselves, did not react or behave until they were stimulated; they were just blanks waiting for stimuli, and then they reacted. That is exactly how it is not. Animals are inquisitive and go out to explore the world. They are seeking what is interesting to them (Nathan, 1997).

What is interesting for a specific patient can be discovered only by trial and error, but a basic condition is that the sensory task should be something that he can do. Another factor promoting the patient's interest and curiosity is his involvement in choosing the sensory task. These and other principles of SRE will be elaborated later, in the context of motivation and the therapeutic relationship.

Variety

Another basic requirement for a successful session of SRE is variety. Sustained attention feeds on change. Our sensory-perceptual systems are geared to detecting change – novel events and movements. Even at the level of the primary sensory receptors, a constant stimulus produces adaptation, and a constantly fixated object 'disappears' (Riggs et al., 1953). Craig reported an illuminating study of the effects of prolonged tactile stimulation, which he undertook in the expectation that 'providing additional stimulation to an area would enhance spatial sensitivity' (Craig, 1992). The results were exactly the opposite. Four young adult volunteers, each wearing vibrators on one arm throughout waking hours, began after a week or two to report strange sensations and were found to make large errors in locating touch, including feeling a single touch in two different locations. These disturbances and a general decline in sensory function persisted for up to 15 weeks after the vibrators were removed. Monotonous, meaningless stimulation, which represents 'noise' rather than information, is therefore not only not beneficial for the restoration of sensory function, but may actually be harmful.

In a session of SRE there should be frequent changes of task, moving between different domains of sensation – such as touch and proprioception – as well as using different parts of the arm, hand and fingers. There should also be frequent breaks for rest. Sensory work is tiring for the patient, even when he is repeating things that he is able to do. Weber, a towering figure in the early attempts to link structure and function in the field of sensation, wrote that 'the senses are fatigued and tired by continuous work, so that we can no longer perceive differences which were formerly noticed very easily and clearly' (Weber, 1834/1978), and he was describing a normal phenomenon. Stroke patients tire easily. The anatomist Brodal, who made a good recovery from stroke, noted that he 'became much more easily tired than previously from mental work', and that 'there was a marked reduction in the powers of concentration' (Brodal, 1973). If the patient tires he will stop concentrating. He therefore needs to have frequent rests, for instance while the therapist puts away equipment or prepares for a different task. The patient also needs to change his position, with help if necessary. Although it is an easily observed phenomenon that the effort to feel something in one's hand brings about a lowering of muscular tension (in contrast to the rise in tension with an effort to move), and there is some evidence that muscle tone is lowered by sensory work (Konno, 1989), the patient may become stiff by staying in one position. After working with his hand on the table, he can change to something that he can do with his hand in his lap or hanging down beside him.

The setting, and the length and frequency of SRE sessions

It is essential that SRE sessions take place in quiet surroundings. A busy therapy department full of other patients is not the right place. Instead, a quiet room should be set aside for it. If this has to be a large room or a place where something else is going on, the patient should sit with his back to the rest of the room. Everything should be done to reduce distracting sounds or sights.

Wynn Parry 'found four ten-minute sessions a day to be of more value than one long session' (Wynn Parry and Salter, 1976). Dellon was also of the opinion that 'frequent short sessions are more productive than longer, less frequent sessions' (Dellon, 1988), and it is clear from his description that he co-opted other staff members, relatives and visitors for this work while the therapist saw the patient only once a week.

These opinions must be respected, and they seem at first sight to be supported by evidence from educational psychology attesting to the benefit of 'distributed practice' – with many short spaced sessions – as opposed to 'massed practice', for successful learning (Smith and Rothkopf, 1984; Glover and Corkhill, 1987). It should, however, be noted that these studies concern schoolchildren and school learning with its emphasis on knowledge, and they are not necessarily relevant to the very different type of skill learning demanded of stroke patients in SRE. It is generally believed, for instance, that 'massed practice is more efficient for simple skills that can be mastered to overlearning with relative ease' (Good and Brophy, 1990), and the overlearning that comes through repetition of a task already mastered is considered to be – both cognitively and neurophysiologically – a process that is different from the learning involved in the initial acquisition of the skill (Krueger, 1929; Pascual-Leone, Grafman and Hallett 1994).

Fitts and Posner, in their pioneer work on skill acquisition, state that 'in the development of most skills, frequent repetition within short periods of time results in a greater depression in performance than the same amount of repetition with more frequent rests' (Fitts and Posner, 1967) and attribute this to declining motivation during continuous performance of a skill. This suggests that even if the patient is succeeding well on a certain task, he should not continue on it too long, but change to another task. Fitts concluded that 'there is no single optimal schedule for all skills, but frequent rest periods seem to facilitate performance'. They also stressed the importance of immediate feedback of results as a strong source of motivation.

In applying the findings on learning in schoolchildren to our present concern, it must be borne in mind that the comparison in the context of schools is between, say, four or five half-hour lessons a week and one block of 2–3 hours, whereas the choice for stroke patients lies between Wynn Parry's four ten-minute sessions throughout the day or one 40-minute session. It is not always feasible to expect the patient to come to the special SRE room more than once a day, and frequent short sessions are not a practical option in the framework of home care or in the case of a patient coming for therapy as an out-patient. But some approximation to the 'little and often' principle can be achieved by encouraging the patient to do whatever sensory 'homework' he and the therapist have decided on several times a day and by involving the patient's relatives in this. At the same time, this is no substitute for regular formal lessons. My own experience has been that most patients find sessions of half an hour to an hour not only possible but even enjoyable, provided the work is taken at a leisurely pace with the right amount of variety and plenty of rests.

Motivation

Closely related to attention, and of no less importance for the success of Sensory Re-education, is the subject of motivation. This section could also have been titled 'hopelessness', 'depression' or 'loss of confidence', because these fairly describe the mood of the majority of patients coming to rehabilitation after stroke, a fact that cannot be ignored by anyone hoping to motivate a stroke patient towards his rehabilitation. 'Somebody who has had a bad stroke will never before have met such a personal disaster to the ego' (Griffith, 1980). The stroke was in most cases unpredictable, a bolt from the blue, and the future is also unpredictable: it may bring death, another stroke or, at best, partial recovery. Goodstein, giving psychiatric consultation to stroke patients during their rehabilitation, wrote that an acute sense of unpredictability and loss of personal control was 'the most distressing psychologic condition reported' (Goodstein, 1983).

Lack of control was the cornerstone of the theory of 'learned helplessness' which Seligman advanced to explain the finding that dogs repeatedly subjected to unavoidable electric shock while restrained by a harness seemed, when released from the harness, to have lost their normal ability to learn how to avoid the shock: they had apparently learned that this was a situation beyond their control (Seligman, 1975). Unavoidable trauma may be expected to produce learned helplessness even more readily in human beings since loss of control for us has the added dimension of projection into the future (Gilbert, 1992), with a long – perhaps endless – prospect of ineffectiveness and helplessness. 'The ominous overtones of what seem to be only two options – sudden death or survival as an invalid – loom heavily for most elderly patients who have had a cerebrovascular accident' (Goodstein, 1983). To the apathy seen in Seligman's traumatized dogs is added the quite rational fear of engaging in any activity that might bring on another stroke. It is interesting to note that some have argued against Seligman's concept of learned helplessness as a non-adaptive, pathopsychological reaction, saying that it may seem counterproductive in the artificial conditions of a laboratory but in nature, where it is found throughout the animal kingdom, it may be a useful reaction for survival: 'showing 'lifelessness' may cause the 'trauma' (e.g. another animal) to go away' (Eisenstein and Carlson, 1997). Some features of mental and emotional disorders are beginning to be interpreted as adaptive responses evolved to deal with the tribulations of life (McGuire and Troisi, 1998), an approach which echoes the ecological interpretation of motor behaviour after stroke discussed in Chapter 4. Perhaps the 'learned helplessness' of a stroke patient would be more appropriately described as 'survival tactics'. If the therapist accepts that there may be a biologically adaptive aspect to the stroke patient's apathy and sometimes even hostility towards therapy, she may be able to gain his confidence and co-operation by listening to him, eliciting and discussing his fears, thereby reaching shared decisions about therapy and his role in it.

The stroke patient's loss of control and helplessness are objective, visible aspects of his predicament. There are other, less visible forces working to sap his confidence and energy, his morale and motivation. Griffith, quoted above, described stroke as a 'disaster to the ego'. One component of this is the drastic loss of dignity, social role and self-esteem, and 'the higher the patient's I.Q. and responsibilities prior to the stroke, the harder the fall' (Griffith, 1980). Inevitably, hospitalization in many ways compounds the stroke's assault on the self. Instead of being able to carry on with life in all its familiar settings, the patient finds himself confined within unfamiliar surroundings and living in a community of people who are total strangers to him. He is like a new boy at boarding school: frail though he is, he has to start 'learning the ropes'. It is perhaps unfair to the humane and dedicated staff of most modern hospitals and rehabilitation centres to quote from Goffman's 'Asylums' in this context (Goffman, 1961) since this book deals, after all, with mental hospitals and other 'total institutions'. However, no one has expressed so strongly some of the unnerving effects of hospitalization which surely add to the low morale of a stroke patient. Here are some passages from Goffman's book.

> Each phase of the member's daily activity is carried on in the immediate company of a large batch of others ... the inmate is never fully alone; he is always within sight and often earshot of someone, if only his fellow inmates.... There are certain bodily comforts significant to the individual that tend to be lost upon entrance to a total institution – for example, a soft bed or quietness at night. Loss of this set of comforts is apt to reflect a loss of self-determination ... the new inpatient finds himself cleanly stripped of many of his accustomed affirmations, satisfactions, and defenses, and is subjected to a rather full set of mortifying experiences: restriction of free movement, communal living, diffuse authority of a whole echelon of people, and so on. Here one begins to learn about the limited extent to which a conception of oneself can be sustained when the usual setting of supports for it are suddenly removed (Goffman, 1961).

Gilbert (1992) chose as the subtitle of his book on depression 'The evolution of powerlessness'. Approaching the subject from the perspective of evolutionary biology, Gilbert related depression in man to the 'depressed' state of a subordinate animal when defeated in the battle for social rank and control or power. His bio-social concept emphasizes the importance of self-esteem to our emotional well-being, with its roots in social control and the sense of belonging. This picture of depression will recall the concept of learned helplessness (Seligman, 1975), with an added social dimension derived from the fact that 'rank is a key social dimension for all social animals' (Gilbert, 1992). Although Gilbert's is essentially a social theory of depression, he gives less attention than one would wish to the effect of calamitous life events, acting through role reversal and loss of self-esteem, in the evolution of depression. In the present context, to the effect of a stroke must be added – in the vast majority of cases – the effects of underlying ageing. Bromley (1966), in his perceptive discussion of motivation and frustration in old age, writes:

> Under conditions of frustration and emotional stress, a person's motivational state becomes strongly focused on the immediate future, concerned with protecting his self-interests and mobilizing his inner resources. During early adult life, presumably, ... motivation towards expanse of the ego predominates ... In later life, however, motivation towards withdrawal, avoidance and substitution predominates, because the person's physical and psychological resources cannot sustain the demands being made upon him. A serious sort of frustration is that engendered by any persistent, stressful, no-solution situation which first elicits violent reactions, such as anger or undirected frenzy, and eventually leads to despair, apathetic resignation or stereotyped pathological responses.

Others have discussed the role of life events and their interaction with vulnerability, lack of social support and other factors in the genesis of depression (Paykel, 1978; Oatley and Boulton, 1985), but a comprehensive study still has to be made of the factors involved in the development of depression in elderly patients who have suffered a serious stroke.

Depression after stroke has been much less studied than neglect and the many other disturbances of attention and awareness described in Chapter 3. This is perhaps because, while attentional disturbances provide a fruitful field for elucidating the brain processes underlying cognitive abilities, we are still far from even starting to study the nature of those underlying emotions and moods. The studies that have been reported suffer from a lack of definition and an unclear distinction between depression as a direct consequence of the brain lesion and depression as a reaction to the stroke. There is therefore considerable contradiction between the findings of different studies. There is, however, a fairly general consensus that depression is common. A comparison between patients coming to rehabilitation one month after stroke and orthopaedic patients admitted at the same time with severe arthritis or hip fracture and matched for physical disability, found 45% of the stroke patients to be depressed compared with only 10% of the orthopaedic patients (Folstein, Maiberger and McHugh, 1977). The authors concluded that 'mood disorder is a more specific complication of stroke than simply a response to the motor disability'. They found the prevalence of depression much higher after right than left hemisphere stroke, but as their diagnosis of depression was based on personal interviews their sample may have underrepresented left hemisphere patients with severe aphasia and possibly depression. A similar exclusion of patients with the severest left hemisphere strokes casts doubt on the conclusion of a recent study which found depression four times more frequent in right hemisphere stroke than in left (MacHale et al., 1998). Another study found depression in one third of 113 stroke patients followed up for 6 months and drew attention to the almost complete lack of treatment (meaning drug treatment) for this depression (Feibel, Berk and Joynt, 1979). Robinson and Price monitored depression over one year in 103 post-stroke patients, also finding depression in one third, two thirds of whom were still depressed 7–8 months later and not receiving treatment for their depression (Robinson and Price, 1982). The clinical symptoms in these depressed patients included 'anxiety, depression, hopelessness, irritability, social withdrawal, ... agitation, loss of interest, and loss of energy'. The prevalence of depression showed no association with neurological symptoms, level of cognitive impairment or degree of disability in daily life activities. Depression, in this study, was markedly commoner in the left hemisphere stroke patients than in the right hemisphere group. Wade and colleagues, who reported depression in 25–30% of stroke survivors at various times during the first year, also found an association with the side of the lesion, but only at three weeks after stroke, when left hemisphere patients had a very much higher frequency of depression (Wade, Legh-Smith and Hewer, 1987).

More recent studies have attempted, with limited success, to distinguish between depression and other emotional disturbances which may occur separately or together with depression. Questioning of participants in the Oxford community stroke project found 'emotionalism' (excessive and uncontrollable crying) in 11–21% of patients, with no significant variation in the prevalence over the first year after stroke (House et al., 1989). These patients also tended to have more general signs of mood disorder and more cognitive problems. A later study from the same project identified 22% of patients followed up for one year after stroke as presenting with psychiatric disorder at some time during the year (House et al., 1991), but noted that most of the small number of patients with persistent psychiatric problems had had these problems before the stroke. These authors came to the conclusion that 'undue emphasis has been placed in the recent literature on major depression as a specific syndrome following stroke', to the neglect of a wide range of milder and commoner emotional disorders such as anxiety, irritability, and social withdrawal. These, which are also common in other patient communities, were especially frequent in the first months after stroke, but reported to decline over the following months. However, a recent 3-year longitudinal study of 'generalized anxiety disorder' in 80 stroke patients (Astrom, 1996) paints a rather different picture: this condition was diagnosed in 28% during the acute stage, and there was no significant decrease in this proportion over the following three years. Major depression was also diagnosed in more than half of these patients. In view of the contradictory findings noted previously about the involvement of the right or left hemisphere, it is interesting that generalized anxiety disorder in the acute stage was found to be associated with lesion of the right hemisphere, whereas anxiety combined with depression was associated with left hemisphere lesion. Anstrom's overall finding of generalized anxiety disorder in 28% of stroke patients is similar to the 27% and 24% found respectively by other studies (Starkstein et al., 1990; Castillo et al., 1993).

Without entering further into the controversies that still surround the subject of emotional disturbances after stroke, it is clear that about one in four stroke patients suffer from acute anxiety, which is likely to persist for months, if not years.

SRE and the anxious patient

This enumeration of the many emotional problems that can beset a stroke patient may seem discouraging for the therapist hoping to embark with him on a course of Sensory Re-education! However, Sensory Re-education is one of the most efficacious paths for aiding the patient to emerge from his low state of mind. As Griffith (1980) writes, 'Stimulation is vital. Unless something can be found to dispel the boredom and inertia in which the patient lives, little can be achieved'. Goffman used a graphic metaphor: 'every total institution can be seen as a kind of dead sea in which little islands of vivid, encapturing activity appear. Such activity can help the individual withstand the psychological stress usually engendered by assaults on the self' (Goffman, 1961).

Since SRE makes little physical demands, it will not be seen as physically threatening, and the quiet dialogue alone with the therapist gives the patient an opportunity to air fears and gain reassurance. If the therapist is fully aware of the factors described above which underlie the patient's apparent lack of motivation, she is already in the position to take on the role of an ally rather than that of a task-master. Her understanding of the patient's problem can perhaps be helped by Maslow's concept of a hierarchy of needs that direct our motivation, which is very relevant to the subject of patient motivation in rehabilitation (Maslow, 1954). This scheme, which states that needs lower in the hierarchy must be satisfied before higher ones, lists in order of priority: 1. physiological needs (sleep, thirst), 2. safety needs (freedom from danger, anxiety or psychological threat), 3. love needs (acceptance from peers, teachers), 4. esteem needs (mastery experiences, confidence in one's ability) and, finally, 5. needs for self-actualization (satisfaction of one's curiosity, creative self-expression). Sensory Re-education seems almost tailored to meet needs 2-4 and even open the way to the possibility of higher self-actualization needs. The patient's needs at the level of physical safety, which as has been stressed, may consciously or unconsciously make him reluctant to participate in physical therapy, are under no threat in the situation of SRE; and the psychological threat of trying to do things which he cannot do, which often pertains in speech therapy (Sadka, 1972), is avoided by the fact that the essence of SRE lies in the patient finding out what he can do. SRE also has another advantage over much of the patient's other therapy: this is that the patient generally has no prior 'correct' experience of sensing things with his hands without looking and therefore has no standard with which to make humiliating comparisons. SRE, as we shall see, is built around success and achievement and, because it concentrates on what the patient **can** do rather than what he cannot do, is an excellent tool for building the self-confidence which must be the basis of successful rehabilitation.

The importance of success

The principle of working from success in SRE receives theoretical support from much of the cognitive psychologists' work on the effect of people's self-perception on their motivation. Particularly relevant is Weiner's study of the role of success and failure in motivation (Weiner, 1966). People with high levels of anxiety tend to fail on difficult tasks, but high-anxiety students did well on the difficult tasks in Weiner's experiments because they were led to believe that they were doing well. Conversely, low-anxiety students – who tend to need difficult challenging tasks for their best performance – did better than expected on the easy tasks because they were led to believe that they were not doing well. This early study suggested that although people with little anxiety are motivated by a perception of failure, high anxiety subjects need to perceive success to be motivated. Failure will occur as well as success in the learning of a skill, but the emphasis for motivating high-anxiety people – like stroke patients – needs to be on success: on ensuring that it occurs, is recognized and praised.

Weiner later incorporated this work into an attributional theory of motivation dealing with the perceived causes of success or failure and their controllability (Weiner, 1986). Success or failure can be attributed to many different causes, and these vary greatly in the degree to which they are perceived as within the person's control. In any situation, people range along a spectrum from those who perceive themselves in control of what happens to those who feel that what happens is beyond their control, being determined by luck or by others. The former are said to have an internal locus of control, the latter an external locus of control (Rotter, 1966). Not surprisingly, students with an internal locus of control tend to get higher grades and achievement scores than those with an external locus of control (Good and Brophy, 1990). More relevant for us, patients with a higher level of perceived control over their recovery have been shown to recover better after severe accidents (Bulman and Wortman, 1977), after spinal cord injury (Shadish, Hickman and Arvick, 1981), and after stroke (Partridge and Johnston, 1989). Locus of control is a dynamic concept: it can vary from situation to situation and change under the influence of the individual's experience. There are many ways in which patients' perception of their control over their recovery can be increased. These include the sharing of knowledge between professionals and patients (Johnston et al., 1992), collaboration in defining problems and planning therapy (Payton, Ozer and Nelson, 1990), and setting meaningful and achievable goals (Kaplan, Atkins and Reinsch, 1984). All three of these ways of increasing patients' sense of control and autonomy are basic principles of the therapeutic relationship in SRE, as described in the next chapter.

Expectations and goals

Another relevant contribution from psychology concerns the subject of expectations and the setting of goals. Feather developed a theory of motivation based on an 'expectancy times value' model (Feather, 1982). This postulates that the effort that people are prepared to put into a task is a product of the degree to which they expect to be able to succeed and the value that they place on the outcome. In other words, we are motivated to do something if we value the outcome and believe that we can achieve it. Conversely, if either factor is absent, there will be no motivation. If a patient does not believe that he can do what the therapist asks of him or 'doesn't see the point of it', he will not be motivated. If the goals of therapy are not determined by the therapist and the patient co-operatively and explicitly, the patient may feel that what the therapist is trying to achieve has little relevance to his personal problems and needs. A number of studies have, in fact, found considerable mismatch between stroke patients and their therapists in their identification of both the goals of the therapy and the degree to which progress has been achieved (Kelman and Willner, 1962; Taylor, 1974; Partridge, 1984; Chiou and Burnett, 1985; Reid and Chesson, 1998). Such a mismatch may be expected to have a very negative effect on the patient's motivation. The patient will be maximally motivated if he believes that he can succeed at what is being demanded of him and if he values the outcome or, in other words, has participated in setting the goal and choosing the task as beneficial for himself. In his social learning theory Bandura stressed the importance for motivation of setting goals that are both proximal and specific and that pose the appropriate amount of challenge (Bandura and Schunk, 1981), and he showed that 'getting students to set goals and make a commitment to try to reach these goals increases their performance'. The motivating effect of setting specific goals is not limited to the field of education, but has been demonstrated in many contexts – in the office, in industry and in laboratory settings, and the effect seems to operate by focusing and directing a person's activity and by spurring him or her to persist to the end (Locke and Latham, 1984).

These are only a small selection of the many rather similar cognitive theories of motivation. Good and Brophy (1990) summarize them well: 'The theories all agree that motivation is optimized when people believe that they are engaging in tasks for their own reasons rather than in response to external pressure, [and] when they see the task as moderately challenging but feel capable of succeeding on it if they invest reasonable effort'.

The method of Sensory Re-education presented here evolved through an ad hoc mixture of intuition and trial and error. It is therefore encouraging to find that its basic approach to the problem of motivating the patient is supported by studies from psychology. These suggest that a stroke patient will be best motivated to take an active part in his own rehabilitation if he expects and experiences success, if he is actively involved in setting specific goals, if he believes that he has some measure of personal control over the situation and if he feels free from physical or psychological threat.

These features of SRE call for a rather special style of interaction between the therapist and the patient. This is described in the next chapter.

Chapter 6
The essentials of Sensory Re-education

The focus on the hand

This book presents a method for re-educating the sensory function of the hand in stroke patient. Why the hand? Sensory deficit after stroke is not limited to the hand or to the upper limb. In fact, sensory loss in the trunk or lower limb contributes to abnormal posture and gait in stroke patients, and this subject will be touched on very briefly in the final chapter.

There are a number of reasons for focusing on the hand. In the first place, the hand is not only a tool – like the leg – but also a sense organ, and its usefulness is totally dependent on its special sensitivity. The hand as a sense organ has often been compared to the eye, and the finger tips likened to the retina's area of maximum visual acuity at the yellow spot – the *macula lutea* (Bell, 1833). Like the eye, the hand provides us with a vital means for exploring the environment. In both the eye and the hand, movement and sensory function are mutually dependent. A large repertoire of independent finger movements serves the hand in its sensory functions, and sensation in turn makes possible the full use of manual dexterity. Both hand and eye are highly mobile structures, not only by virtue of their delicate intrinsic musculature but also through their attachment to chains of anatomical links with many degrees of freedom. Although the hand, unlike the eye, does not have a whole lobe of the cerebral hemisphere devoted to its input, it monopolizes a disproportionately large part of the sensory cortex. Compared with the much smaller foot area, which lies deep in the cleft between the two hemispheres, the hand's cortical representation is both large and relatively accessible. The hand has therefore been the preferred site for neurophysiologists studying the effects of experience – injury or training – on the functional organization of the cortex, so that there is a rich theoretical basis on which to build a therapeutic approach to the problem of sensory loss in the hand.

An additional reason for focusing on the hand is that it is particularly vulnerable to learned non-use. As a result of the paramount place of sensation in the usefulness of the hand, a patient with inadequate sensation in the hand is unlikely to use it, whatever its motor potential. The other hand will take over all the fine tasks of everyday life, and the patient will behave much like an upper limb amputee or someone with one arm in a sling. Fine sensation plays a vastly less important part in modern man's use of his feet, and sensory deficit in the foot or leg will not prevent walking and is never the only reason for a stroke patient's failure to walk. The insensate hand is therefore more prey to learned non-use than the insensate leg.

The final reason for our focus, and a very cogent one, is that the functional recovery of the hand and upper limb after stroke tends to be much poorer than that of the lower limb (Olsen, 1989). The hand seems to be specially vulnerable in stroke, both as regards the primary lesion and at the levels of impairment and disability, and this is only partly due to the detrimental effects of learned non-use. This heightened vulnerability could be related to the fact that the special manipulative functions of the human hand are – in evolutionary terms – a relatively recent acquisition, and they are learned only gradually throughout childhood, long after the child can walk. An alternative, more prosaic explanation of the upper and lower limbs' disparate records for functional recovery could be that this is a 'loaded' comparison: the lower limb is considered to be functional if the patient can walk, while the upper limb is judged on doing up buttons and shoe-laces! Whatever the explanation, the fact is that a large number of stroke survivors achieve a reasonable level of mobility but are left with a more or less useless hand.

Sensory Re-education therefore focuses on the hand, a) because of the hand's special importance as a sense organ, b) because sensation is vital for fine manual dexterity, and c) because the hand tends to be especially incapacitated by stroke. The 'rehabilitated' stroke patient with a useless hand presents a challenge that demands an answer.

The therapeutic relationship

Therapists working in stroke rehabilitation spend most of their time examining and treating patients. The method of Sensory Re-education (SRE) presented in this book is a different kind of activity, unlike either examining or treating. As therapists often find the transition to SRE a difficult one, it is important to devote some consideration to the nature of this transition and to the habits of thought, the ways of working and, above all, the style of interaction with the patient that need to be developed for SRE.

Looking for abilities rather than disabilities

SRE is essentially a process in which the patient learns with the therapist's help to discover and use whatever somatic sensations are available to him and in whatever reduced or distorted form they may 'filter through'. SRE, like any learning process, requires motivation and achievement, the patient's motivation leading to achievement and this then feeding his motivation. The focus is therefore on what the patient *can* do, a point that cannot be overemphasized. The habit of looking for 'signs and symptoms' is strongly entrenched in all medical professionals, and a therapist starting to use SRE will tend to revert to the testing situation in which the patient's performance is, as it were, driven inexorably towards failure. If he succeeds in one task, he is given a harder one until the limit of his abilities is reached. This process has a legitimate place in testing sensation, as in testing other functions, but it has no place in SRE. In SRE, when the patient succeeds in a task, he should be encouraged to repeat it several times before exploring related tasks that may now be possible with this new found skill. Repetition, in Bernstein's sense of solving the problem in increasingly efficient ways (Bernstein, 1967), is an essential part of learning, and a sensory task that is difficult and uncertain at first becomes easy and assured with practice. Repetition of the new skill brings the patient to the final 'autonomous' phase in Fitts' model of skill learning, in which performance becomes 'less directly subject to cognitive control', more rapid and more efficient (Fitts and Posner, 1967).

Collaboration

The process of working with – rather than on – the patient is another feature in which SRE differs from treatment. A large part of traditional therapy for stroke patients consists of working *on* the patient, moving and manipulating him to produce desired reactions, whether these are postural responses or a decrease in spasticity. His is a relatively passive role, and it is not necessary that he understand either the methods or the immediate aims of the therapy that he is receiving. As already mentioned, there may even be considerable mismatch between the treatment goals of patients and their therapists. Skilled handling of a passive patient may have a rational basis in therapy aimed at eliciting motor responses, but from our review of the neurophysiological literature it is clearly inappropriate for re-educating sensory function.

Sharing knowledge

Unlike the traditional therapist working on a patient's motor behaviour, the SRE therapist is from the start totally dependent on the patient for knowing what is going on in his 'sensorium'. Only the patient knows what he feels, and the therapist's job is to enter into his inner sensory world so that she can help to guide him and direct him there. SRE is a collaborative activity, involving mutual sharing of knowledge and the sharing of control and responsibility.

SRE begins with the therapist sharing her knowledge with the patient. Stroke patients can be surprisingly unaware of the severity of their condition (Grotta and Bratina, 1995), and patients with sensory loss are specially unlikely to be aware of this, even if they do not suffer from some form of neglect or anosognosia. Levine has pointed out that sensory loss is not phenomenally immediate: it has to be discovered – by self-observation and inference or by having it demonstrated (Levine, 1990). Patients with sensory loss often describe their hand as 'heavy', 'cold' or just 'useless' and seldom realize that they cannot feel the hand or feel anything with it. They are even less aware of sensory deficit in other parts of the body. Few healthy people have ever given a thought to the sensory systems involved in their simplest activities, and stroke patients are seldom aware that sensation plays any part in their disabilities. The therapist should explain to the patient that the control of movement requires sensation, reminding him for instance how difficult it is to drink or whistle after a purely sensory injection at the dentist. She should show him that part of the 'uselessness' of his hand comes from his being unable to know – without looking – where his hand is or to feel things that she puts in his hand. SRE is presented to him as a method by which, with the therapist's help, he will learn to feel with his hand, like a blind person learning to read Braille with his finger tips. The therapist should stress that the work will demand from him both a lot of concentration and constant practice, but that it has a good chance of helping him recover some of the use of his hand.

Sharing control

The patient should be as much in control of his own sensory re-education as possible. Whenever practicable during SRE sessions he should be encouraged to choose what he thinks he can do, rather than having the choice made for him by the therapist. For instance, he may be asked to choose two or three objects which he thinks he may be able to distinguish by touch. After he has chosen them, the therapists asks him to say what the differences are between them – in shape, weight, consistency and the like – which he thinks he can use as clues to help him guess which of them he has in his hand. In this way he participates in developing a plan of action for the sensory task ahead of him. This 'thinking about' the objects or tasks is part of the tactics of perception which he is learning and which will be discussed more fully later. He should be encouraged to think up sensory tasks which he can practise by himself. Many of the methods and tools of SRE were, in fact, contributed by patients.

In summary, SRE is a collaboration between therapist and patient in which the therapist works with – rather than on – the patient. The work focuses on identifying and enlarging the patient's sensory abilities, rather than on the traditional medical categorization of pathology and disability: in other words, on what the patient can do rather than on what he cannot do. Knowledge is shared, and explicit and immediate goals are determined in collaboration. The patient takes the initiative as much as possible in running the session, as well as being responsible for practice and progress between sessions. The patient's active participation – in the best case, his enthusiastic involvement – is a major force in his sensory recovery.

The protocol for a sensory task

Approaching the task, or the tactics of perception

A new sensory task does not begin with the therapist testing the patient. Instead, the task starts with the patient and the therapist discussing it together and the patient trying it out with his good hand. For instance, today the patient thinks that he may be able to distinguish between two wooden shapes, one square in outline, the other triangular.

> *'What are the differences you think you can feel?'*
> 'Well, the triangle has three corners, the square has four.'
> *'What else?'*
> 'I think the corners of the triangle feel sharper, more pointed.' (He closes his eyes and the therapist puts the triangle in his good hand).
> 'Of course, this is a triangle, I can tell by the sharpness of the corners without counting them.'

Note that the 'sharpness of the corners' is a reliable diagnostic attribute only for the equilateral triangle which he has in his hand. Using a right-angle triangle could lead to mistaking it for a square. This point can be raised later if the patient reaches such a sophisticated level of sensory discrimination.

This sort of analysis, which played such a large part in the sensory rehabilitation described by Leont'ev and Zaporozhets, serves to focus the patient's complete attention on the task and prepare him for learning to do it with his affected hand. It can be done while looking at the object, while handling it with the good hand with eyes shut, and with the affected hand with eyes open or shut. Two studies reporting reduced reaction time to tactile stimuli when the eyes are directed to the stimulus suggest that directing the gaze – even with eyes shut – towards the hand that is palpating the object is likely to enhance its sensory performance (Honoré, Bourdeaud'hui and Sparrow, 1989; Pierson et al., 1991).

These three 'modes of discourse' – discussing, looking and feeling with the good hand – use different areas of the brain, and their relative import-ance as paths to learning varies enormously, both for different tasks and for different people. Some people learn 'cognitively', some by watching, some by doing, and the three activities play different roles in different activities. When we add to the normal range of people's styles and habits the almost infinite variety of brain damage that can result from a stroke, we get some idea of the multiplicity of paths that must be explored for the re-education of sensory function after stroke. The categorical statement that every new sensory task begins with these three activities must, therefore, be modified. These are the three basic approaches available. Which, and in what order or combination to use them, depends on the task and on the patient.

The use of the good hand

Clearly, a new sensory task will start with some sort of discussion and inspection of the task and its tools. It should then proceed to experiencing the task with the good hand. Working with the good hand is important in the first place for getting the patient used to exploring his sensations with his eyes shut. It is even more important for helping him to become aware of his tactics of perception, as illustrated in the example of the triangle and the square. Our recognition of a common object held in the hand is so rapid that we have named the object before we can begin to say how we did it. Quite a lot of time needs to be spent working with the good hand in order to clarify this process of recognition sufficiently for teaching it to the affected hand. For example, when the patient – using his good hand – makes an apparently instantaneous differentiation between a metal tool and a sponge, does the clue come from the weight (hefting it), the consist-ency (squeezing it), the shape (feeling the outline), temperature, or what? As tactile training has recently been shown to transfer from one hand to the other hand (Sathian and Zangaladze, 1997), this preliminary work with the good hand may help to 'prime' the other hand. When the patient passes on to the affected hand, it is often advisable for him to start with his eyes open, looking at his hand and naming the sensory clues, and only then try to repeat this with his eyes closed.

This emphasis on the patient using his good hand to teach his affected hand rests not only on personal experience, but on a variety of neurophysio-logical studies attesting to bilateral activity in the brain during one-handed activity. It was for long thought that the cortical sensory representation of the hand and fingers was limited to the contralateral hemisphere (Jones and Powell, 1969), but widespread and complex bilateral representations have recently been demonstrated (Iwamura, Iriki and Tanaka, 1994; Burton et al., 1997). One line of evidence for the involvement of both hemispheres during single-handed activity comes from electromyography (EMG). Many years ago, what was called 'motor irradiation' (Cernacek, 1961) was described in healthy adults in the form of EMG activity from symmetrical muscles on the side opposite to a voluntarily contracting muscle in healthy adults. Visible associated movements or 'mirror movements' occur normally in young children (Wolff, Gunnoe and Cohen, 1983; Lazarus and Todor, 1987) and persist in many subjects with neurological disorders (Abercrombie, Lindon and Tyson, 1964). They also occur in hemiplegic patients after stroke (Walshe, 1923), especially when there is spasticity. Green (1967) studied mirror movements and EMG recordings in stroke patients and found that a strong flexion of the unaffected hand or elbow was regularly followed by EMG activity – and often visible contraction – in the equivalent muscles on the affected arm; the stronger the voluntary contraction, the shorter the delay.

The other line of evidence for a potential contribution of both sides of the brain to the performance of one-handed tasks comes from PET studies showing ipsilateral brain activity in recovered stroke patients performing tasks with their formerly paralysed hands. This work was described in Chapter 4. Here it is interesting to add that some of these patients showed slight mirror movements in the *unaffected* hand: in other words, in the hand which, though not actively engaged in the activity, is the one normally controlled by the hemisphere that had apparently taken over some control of the affected hand (Weiller et al., 1992; Weiller et al., 1993; Weder et al., 1994).

Summary

This and the previous chapters have dealt with many subjects and drawn quite eclectically on contributions from a wide range of disciplines. It may be helpful to summarize the basic principles of Sensory Re-education.

1. The focus on the hand

Though sensory loss after stroke is not limited to the hand, the hand is the main target for SRE. This is because its usefulness is intimately tied up with its sensory powers, without adequate sensation it is especially prey to learned non-use, and the 'rehabilitated' stroke patient with a useless hand is a distressingly common phenomenon.

2. Attention and motivation

Therapy for stroke patients needs to be active and interesting if it is to tap the brain's potential for functional reorganization. At the same time, account must be taken of the fact that stroke patients are often elderly and anxious and reluctant to comply with any demands that may bring on another stroke. Sensory Re-education is a quiet, non-threatening collaboration between therapist and patient in which she helps him to discover his abilities, rather than his disabilities. The experience of success – of being able to do something – is the key to engaging his interest, to motivating him to take an active part in his recovery and to building the self-confidence which is the basis of rehabilitation.

3. Conducting a session of SRE

SRE must be carried out in a quiet place, with a minimum of distraction. The work concentrates on sensory tasks that the patient *can* do, that he enjoys doing and that he participates in choosing. Variety is essential, including varying sensory modalities, varying the area of the hand or arm and varying the position of the patient's arm. He should also have frequent rests. With plenty of variety and rest, most patients can enjoy sessions of three-quarters of an hour to one hour.

Each new sensory task begins with the therapist and the patient discussing it and the patient exploring it with his good hand. What does it feel like? How does he do it? What are the salient clues that he will have to look for when he uses his other hand? He then tries it out with his affected hand, first with his eyes open and then with eyes closed. The session ends with the patient choosing tasks and equipment for 'homework' that he can do alone or with the help of friends and relatives, until his next meeting with the therapist.

Chapter 7
The curriculum I

How to use the curriculum

This and the following chapter describe lessons for the re-education of stroke patients in the sensory functions of the hand. The lessons are intended to be used both as described and as models from which to develop other ways of re-educating sensation.

Much thought went into deciding how to arrange this curriculum. It would seem logical to arrange the lessons in order from the easiest to the most difficult, rather like graded exercises for playing the piano or a 'Teach yourself Spanish' book. However, patients vary so much in their sensory deficits and sensory abilities that what is easy for one patient may be difficult for another, and there is no universal order of difficulty. Additionally, in line with the cardinal principle that SRE must be interesting if it is to succeed, patients often fail at an easy sensory task but succeed at one that seems much harder, simply because it catches their interest.

An alternative order would be an anatomical one – from proximal to distal. This would start with sensory functions around the shoulder and upper arm and progress to the forearm and hand. This order has a certain logic since sensation is often less affected in the proximal parts than in the hand, and a patient's interest in SRE can sometimes be first aroused by finding, for instance, that he can recognize a letter traced on his arm which he cannot even feel on the palm of his hand, or that he can feel whether his elbow is straight or flexed before he can do this for his fingers. But here again, this is far from universal, and the very common painful hemiplegic shoulder (Teasell and Gillen, 1993) argues against starting in this area.

A third way, and the one used here, is to adopt the framework of everyday neurology and group the lessons roughly in the order that neurologists use when they examine sensation. They traditionally examine, in this order: sensitivity to touch, pain and temperature, sense of position and passive movement, sensitivity to vibration, two-point discrimination, and finally appreciation of form or stereognosis (Brain, 1933). As a classification of somatic sensory function this list is a sort of cocktail made up of sensory modalities and perceptual functions: sensory modalities traditionally associated with structural components of the peripheral nervous system, and perceptual functions which can be differentiated subjectively and may be dissociated in patients with central lesions. However, it is a familiar and time-honoured way of thinking about sensory function, and it suggests a way of dividing the field to form a curriculum for Sensory Re-education. The neurological examination first tests some basic exteroceptive functions, notably touch, then proprioceptive functions, and finally the derived functions of two-point discrimination and stereognosis.

Following this scheme, SRE is presented as a curriculum comprising three main subjects: touch, proprioception and object recognition. The first two subjects, touch and proprioception, cover the two somatic sources of information available to us: the external, cutaneous source through our contact with objects, and the internal source, from the deep receptors in the joints, muscles and other tissues. Apart from the organs of special sense, these two sources provide us with all that we know about ourselves and our environment, and they are essential for our interaction with it.

While this classical distinction between exteroception and proprioception furnishes a useful framework for presenting SRE, they blend together inextricably in the sensory activities of daily life. Proprioception – although meaning literally sensation about oneself – is an essential tool for the hand's exploration of the environment, and 'exteroceptors' in the skin make their contribution to proprioception and to our body image. Together they form what Gibson dubbed the 'haptic system', as 'the perceptual system by which animals and men are literally in touch with the environment' (Gibson, 1966). The fusion of exteroception and proprioception is expressed in the curriculum's third subject, which comprises lessons in the main sensory function of the hand, namely the examination and recognition of objects, activities which use both externally and internally derived information.

The three parts of the curriculum – touch, proprioception, and object recognition – should be seen as subjects to be taught concurrently, like the three R's in childhood. It cannot be stressed enough that the curriculum is merely a practical way to organize SRE on paper, and that the choice and order of lessons for an individual patient must be determined by only one consideration, and that is the patient's abilities. For instance, with a patient who has very poor sensation and low expectations, it is often inadvisable to start with lessons in touch, which may be too 'academic' for him, but rather with a gross recognition task like distinguishing between a lead dumb-bell and a sponge: this is on the principle that the patient must succeed.

Secondly, the lessons presented do not have to be 'covered' or completed. Each patient will start at a different place and will need and benefit from different lessons. Each session should include various types of work, using a number of different lessons from the three main subjects.

The curriculum aims to give a very full description of the lessons, with live examples and illustrations where they can help. At the same time, the purpose of this book is not to offer yet another collection of recipes ('Well-tried favourites') for stroke rehabilitation, but to present a method for sensory re-education which has been shown to be effective and which has a rational foundation in what is known about sensory function and neuro-plasticity. Many of the lessons are therefore accompanied by quite lengthy discussions of relevant scientific findings and their application to SRE.

Lessons in touch

Touch is the first sense to develop: already in the 11-week human foetus, the palms of the hands respond to touch (Humphrey, 1964). Its primacy among senses is reflected in the wide use which we make of adjectives derived from touch to describe qualities of other senses, as in a warm colour, a dull sound, a sharp taste (Williams, 1976). The curriculum there-fore opens with lessons in touch. These range from the simple to the complex, but such is the importance of the patient's attention and curiosity that he may succeed in what seems a complex, but interesting touch task while failing in an apparently simple but less interesting one. The advice against a slavish adherence to the order of the curriculum is therefore to be borne in mind.

For the simple lessons in touch, the therapist uses something pointed but sufficiently blunt not to cause pain or discomfort. She can use her own finger or the blunt end of a pencil or the handle of a teaspoon, noting only that the cold metal may either be felt more easily than the wood or it may produce an unpleasant sensation. Touch on the plegic arm should be firm and maintained, with long intervals between one touch and the next, because sensory processing is likely to be slow, and there is often persis-tence of an impression after the stimulation has ceased (Holmes, 1927; Karp, Belmont and Birch, 1971).

Lesson 1: How many points?

The lesson starts with the good arm: 'I'm going to touch your arm a number of times, starting near the shoulder and going down. Count the touches out loud as you feel them ... Yes, there were three. How can you tell whether a touch is above the elbow or below it? Is it easier to do this with your elbow bent? Let's see.' This is then repeated with the plegic arm, if necessary with the patient first watching the therapist touching his arm, then without looking. 'Here is a touch high up, near your shoulder. This one is on your forearm. I'll start again at the top. Count aloud and see if you can feel when I get below your elbow' (Fig 7.1).

Lesson 2: Lines

'I'm going to trace a line down your arm' (slowly and firmly). 'Try to feel that it goes down, not up... This is a line going up. Now tell me which direction this line goes, up or down. Is it on your upper arm or forearm? .... To make this a bit more interesting, sometimes I'll draw a wavy line, like this. Tell me if this is straight or wavy.... Now I'll draw a number of lines side by side. Try to tell how many lines there are.'

These and similar exercises in simple touch can also be done on the back of the hand, the palm or the fingers. They are not very interesting, and their main use is that they may serve to show a very impaired and despondent patient that his 'useless' arm is alive and bringing him information. The same aim can be achieved in a more interesting way by tracing numbers or letters.

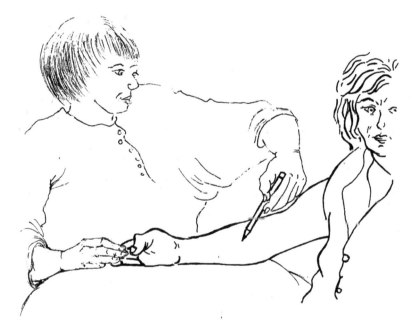

Figure 7.1 How many points?

Lesson 3: Letters

The therapist can ask the patient to choose two or three letters which he thinks sufficiently distinct for him to recognize when they are traced on his arm or hand. Alternately, she can use the letters in Figure 7.2 which have been derived from a very thorough study of the tactile recognition of letters (Vega-Bermudez, Johnson and Hsiao, 1991). The figure shows pairs made up of letters which these authors reported to be the easiest to identify (ILOUW), together with the letter S, which they found to be the most frequently confused with other letters (though not with those in Figure 7.2). Cards can be prepared with two or three of these letters for the patient to look at, or the therapist can write letters in front of the patient, or she can use this figure and cover up the irrelevant parts. She traces them on the patient's good arm or hand. 'Try to define how you know whether I'm writing I, L or O.' The patient might reply, 'The I is just a straight line; I feel the break at the corner in the L as well as the change of direction, whereas the O goes down and up but continuously, without a break.' Changing to the plegic arm, 'Feel that this is just a simple straight line; it is an I. Now this – the L – is essentially two lines, this one down, then a change of direction, and here's the second line to the side. OK? Here's the O. Now I'll do these three letters in a different order. See if you can recognize them.'

In the lessons described up to now, the patient has been passive: no movement has been required of him. But as we move further into the curriculum, we shall find him participating more actively. The effect of movement on sensation is so important and complex a subject that it

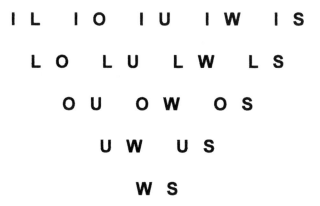

Figure 7.2 Letters for tactile recognition.

cannot be slipped into SRE in this casual fashion. Does movement enhance sensory function? Does it matter whether the patient actively moves his hand over an object or the object is moved over the patient's hand? It may come as a surprise to learn that there are still no unequivocal answers to these questions. However, what is known has a bearing on SRE and merits interrupting the curriculum for a brief review.

Touch and movement

Weber, in his great work on touch, stated that 'the touch-sense is much improved by voluntary movement' (Weber, 1834/1978), and Katz – another author of a weighty German treatise on touch – echoed this: 'movement is well-nigh as indispensable to touch as light is to vision' (Katz, 1925/1989). Gibson raised this view almost to the level of dogma, both by his very influential view of sensory-perceptual systems as active seekers of information (Gibson, 1966) and by his much-quoted demonstration that people are better at discriminating two-dimensional forms (cookie-cutters) when allowed to handle them than when the objects are pressed on their passive palms (Gibson, 1962). However, movement is clearly not the only factor involved in this comparison, because actively manipulating an object provides information both from proprioceptors and from the fingers, which is not available when the object rests on the subject's passive palm. Since Gibson's time, a number of studies under more controlled conditions seem to have established that, while sensory discrimination is enhanced by movement between hand and object, passive touch of a moving object is as informative as active, moving touch of a stationary object.

At first sight it is hard to accept this conclusion. Can we really judge the thickness of paper or the quality of cloth just as well by pulling it through static fingers as by rubbing it between fingers and thumb? And when working with a stroke patient, is the therapist's manipulation of an object or material in his paralysed hand really as adequate for sensory discrimination as his own active exploration would be? The explanation for the paradoxical results of these studies becomes clear from a perusal of the methods used to cut out all possible 'extraneous' differences between the active and the passive situations. In perhaps the most interesting study (Vega-Bermudez, Johnson and Hsiao, 1991), the speed and accuracy with which capital letters are recognized were found to be the same whether a rotating drum passed a letter repeatedly from right to left across the subject's fixed finger pad or the subject made smooth left-to-right horizontal movements of his finger over the letter. This, in the first place, is not the sort of real-life task in which one habitually feels with one's finger-tips. If, however, you can lay your hands on a book with the title embossed on the binding and try to identify the letters with your finger, you will find that you make a great variety of movements, most of them circular or up and down, with small pauses in between; and if you keep your finger still and move the book, the most helpful movement is circular rather than side-to-side. This is not to cast doubt on the experimental findings, but to suggest that a rigid experimental protocol can tell us little about the contribution of movement to touch in a real life situation when the movement is both seeking information and guided by information.

A more serious doubt about the contribution of movement to the sense of touch comes from the discovery that sensory input to the brain, far from being enhanced during movement, is actually suppressed. This surprising observation was reported at about the same time for vision and for touch. We shift our gaze by rapid eye movements (saccades) between one point of fixation and the next, and the transmission of visual input is blocked at a subcortical station during these saccades (Adey and Noda, 1973). Similarly, during movement of, say, a finger the transmission of sensory input from the finger is suppressed at all relay stations up to the cortex (Ghez and Pisa, 1972; Coulter, 1974). This suppression, often termed 'gating', occurs – though to a smaller degree – during passive as well as active movement, and in man as well as in animals (Papakostopoulos, Cooper and Crow, 1975). The faster the movement, the greater the suppression of input to the cortex, and this suppression affects neighbouring fingers as well as the moving finger (Rushton, Rothwell and Craggs, 1981). It starts before the EMG signs of muscle activation, so that it is not produced by feedback from the movement, and it occurs whether the muscle produces a movement or an isometric (static) contraction (Jiang, Lamarre and Chapman, 1990).

It seems wise to suppress the transmission of visual information while glancing from one point to another, as the scene in between is of little interest. But it is hard to see anything but biological disadvantages to cutting off the flow of information while one is engaged in doing something! Here again, the paradox seems to a large extent to result from using stimuli that have no behavioural relevance. In the experiments of Jiang and colleagues, 20 millisecond air-puffs were delivered to a monkey's arm while he performed the elbow movements in which he had been trained and for which he received drops of juice (Jiang, Lamarre and Chapman, 1990). The air-puffs, which might have attracted his attention while resting, were clearly just a distraction when he bent his elbow for a sip of juice, and in this situation they produced much smaller cortical responses. For behaviourally relevant stimuli there seems to be less suppression. For instance, making voluntary muscle contractions has no effect on subjects' threshold or perception of intensity for heat or pain (Feine et al., 1990), and some of the suppression of cortical input from the paws of rats during treadmill walking does not occur when the rats are exploring and walking freely (Chapin and Woodward, 1982). Transmission of a stimulus that is normally suppressed during movement is actually enhanced if the stimulus serves as a go cue for moving (Hyvarinen, Poranen and Jokinen, 1980). Suppression of input thus seems to be highly selective and better described as 'gating'. Studies of activity in different parts of the sensory cortex show that while as much as 50% of the input to the primary sensory cortex may be suppressed during movement, the remaining input undergoes enhanced transmission to the secondary sensory cortex and other areas (Huttunen et al., 1996). In short, the gating of sensory input during movement should perhaps be seen as part of a neural mechanism of selective attention by which 'information of interest for the animal is enhanced while the rest is suppressed' (Chapman, 1994).

What practical suggestions for lessons in touch can we derive from the still controversial data on the contribution of movement to sensation? In the first place, voluntary movement is not essential for sensation; a lot can be done with skilled passive movement, and a severely paralysed patient need not be considered too impaired for sensory re-education. In the second place, the selective gating of sensory input during movement by which 'information of interest ... is enhanced while the rest is suppressed' (Chapman, 1994) provides additional confirmation for the principle that the core process in SRE must be guiding the patient to look for and select what is relevant out of the whole barrage of sensory information. This has already been stated in a number of different contexts as studies in neurophysiology and psychology led again and again to the conclusion that neuroplasticity, functional recovery and learning can only be generated by demands or challenges that are interesting or in some way significant for the organism. The selective gating of sensory input during movement provides a close-up view of part of the neural mechanics of selective attention.

Turning to the actual movements that people make with their hands when exploring materials or objects by touch, these have been studied in great detail by Lederman and Klatzky (1990) who described a number of rather stereotyped 'exploratory procedures' related to the diagnostic attribute being examined. They also reported the frequency with which attributes such as shape, size and texture, formed the main diagnostic attribute for identifying a long list of common objects. These studies are a rich source of information for SRE and will be referred to frequently as we continue the lessons in touch.

Lesson 4: Discrimination of texture

When without looking we identify a common object held in the hand, one of the features which contributes to this process is the texture of the object. The object's size is used about as often as its texture, and only shape surpasses these two in the frequency with which it is used for the tactile recognition of common objects (Lederman and Klatzky, 1990). Texture discrimination is therefore an important element in object recognition, and as such it will figure later in the section devoted to that subject. At the same time, when used on its own instead of as one of many diagnostic properties of an object, texture can provide a useful medium for practising and improving sensitivity to touch. Lessons in texture discrimination also spur the patient to move and to participate more actively than in the lessons described up to now.

The following is a list of objects or materials that can be used, their texture ranging from rough to smooth:

Stiff clothes-brush
Basket
Plastic grid
Corrugated cardboard
Coarse sandpaper
Corduroy
Carpet, rug
Sheepskin
Hessian, sacking
Page of Braille
Fine sandpaper
Cotton
Velvet
Silk
Glass

A longer list could have provided finer grades of texture, but even these are too fine for many stroke patients engaged in SRE. The aim is simply to provide a list from which materials can be chosen that are appropriate to each patient's abilities.

For testing texture discrimination, materials are often mounted on square pieces of plywood, but for teaching it is better to use them in their normal state in sizes that can be easily handled. As in other lessons, the patient surveys them and chooses the ones he thinks he may be able to distinguish. Alternately, the therapist can choose materials which she thinks will guarantee success. A patient might even have to begin with becoming quite certain about differentiating between the bristles of a clothes brush and a glass surface before progressing to, say, a basket and a sheepskin, and thence to more than two materials and to more similar materials. As in other lessons, the therapist encourages the patient to pick out the distinct-ive characteristics of the materials as he looks at them and handles them with his good hand. Corrugated cardboard, for instance, has longitudinal ridges of constant height; the basket also has more or less parallel ridges but their varying height gives the finger the feeling of an undulating surface, whereas the plastic grid has a regular crosshatch of ridges at right-angles to each other.

Comparing two or more textures is a good method for teaching texture discrimination for most patients, but not for all. Henry Head (whom – the reader will have noted – I find an unrivaled source of clinical observations and wisdom) differentiated between two types of disturbed texture discrimination, one produced by defective cortical processing of adequate sensory input, the other related to deficits in the sense of touch (Head, 1918). These two disturbances can occur together but Head found them dissociated in a number of his patients. If textures cannot be named although threshold and location of touch are normal, we are dealing with an agnosia. One such patient of Head's correctly described a piece of silk as 'smooth, silky' but could not identify it as silk: 'It was not ... the smooth-ness and roughness that were not appreciated, but the essential difference which enables us to give each textile material its specific name'. By contrast, patients with poor recognition of textures associated with deficient sense of touch but no agnosia 'usually attempt to name the stuff placed in their hands; but they frequently add some explanation of the difficulty they recognize in determining the character of the material.' The therapist should be on the look out for the contribution of agnosia in a patient who does well in other touch lessons but finds it hard to name textures. For such a patient, less emphasis should be placed on comparing textures and more on naming individual materials. The importance of naming in SRE will be discussed more fully in the next chapter in the context of object recognition.

If the patient has so little power of voluntary movement that he cannot move his hand over the materials, the therapist should watch very carefully how he moves his good hand over the material when he examines it and try to reproduce this when she moves his plegic hand over it. The typical movement for examining texture is a repetitive lateral shearing motion along a surface (Lederman and Klatzky, 1990). Apart from the type of movement made, an important feature of all exploratory procedures which does not seem to have been studied is that movement is typically arrested during shorter or longer pauses: the subject stops moving his fingers, pauses, and then embarks on a different movement. During such a pause, he often frowns as though thinking 'What is it?' or 'What shall I do next?' (such a pause is illustrated in Figure 7.3). At a neurophysiological level, the pause may serve to lift the suppression of sensory input before imposing a new pattern of sensory gating for the next attack on the task. R.S. Johansson (1996) found that sensory information 'intervenes intermittently' during active manipulation of an object. Whatever the function of these pauses, it is important to observe them whilst the patient feels with his good hand and then try to reproduce them when moving his affected hand. The padded roller skate illustrated in Figure 7.4 has proved a very useful support for the patient's forearm which allows the therapist to hold his hand around the knuckles as she moves it over the material which she holds in her other hand. Even if the patient has some control over movement, he may not produce the same exploratory procedures used by his good hand. He can relearn these tactics by watching his hands, sequentially or simultaneously, as he feels materials with them. The therapist should draw his attention to the momentary pauses as well as to the movements he makes with his good hand.

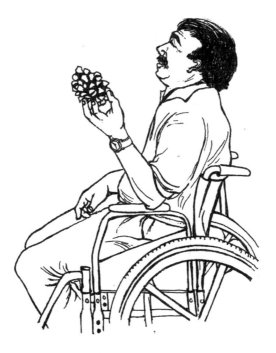

Figure 7.3 A pause during sensory discrimination.

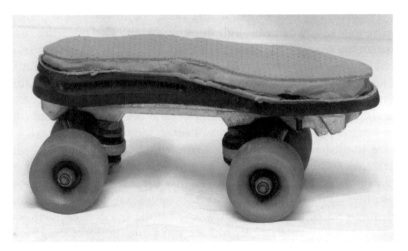

Figure 7.4 The padded roller-skate.

Lesson 5: Identification of fingers

A stroke patient may be able to identify his thumb when it is touched, but no other fingers, or his thumb and little finger but none of the fingers in between. There are also patients who can identify the thumb and index finger and have quite good sensation in them, but lack sensory discrimination on the ulnar side of the hand (and usually in the wrist and forearm also). A more serious disturbance, known as Gerstmann's syndrome (Gerstmann, 1940) is sometimes seen in patients with stroke affecting the right parietal lobe and causing finger agnosia accompanied by right–left confusion and widespread cognitive disturbance. These patients have problems distinguishing not only between their own fingers of either hand but also between the observer's fingers.

Discrimination between the fingers is vital for recognizing objects by touch and for manipulating them. Its re-education needs a lot of imaginative work, especially if there is an agnostic component in the problem. For some patients the subject can best be approached through the lessons described later in the sections on proprioception and the recognition of objects and their qualities, but some suggestions are included here for teaching finger identification directly through touching and moving them.

First, however, it is appropriate to review what is known about finger identification. Many years ago, Halnan and Wright reported a fascinating study of Cambridge University students' location of touch on their fingers and toes (Halnan and Wright, 1960). Their paper highlights the relative uncertainty that people have in locating touch on their middle – second, third and fourth – fingers and toes, as opposed to their greater certainty and accuracy for the thumb and big toe and the little finger and fifth toe. It also provides insight into the methods that people use to help them decide which finger or toe has been touched, because the authors believed that 'the subjective findings in experiments on tactile localization are at least of equal value with the numerical results' and reported their subjects' comments very fully. The following are some of the comments that can be instructive for SRE.

Many of the students used after-effects to help them. Thus, 'If you give it a good dig it lasts longer and you can be more sure.' And, 'There is a sharp feeling first, then a gradual dying-away. It is easier to tell from the after-impression than from the initial,' or 'I now realize the previous one was 7 [radial side of ring finger] because I can still feel it as you touch 5 [radial side of third finger].' The students made fewer errors if they were allowed to move their fingers after being touched. After an experiment in which movement was not allowed, one subject said, 'I kept thinking – if only I could move, I could be absolutely certain,' and when movement was allowed this often led to correcting a previous wrong localization. In some experiments subjects were told to open their eyes and look at their fingers after being touched, and this improved their accuracy, especially for identifying toes. As one student said, 'I was surprised to find how much easier it was to tell, when I looked at my feet. I could sense the position of the stimulus but didn't know which toe was there until I looked.' The authors quote older authorities' reports that directing one's gaze to the point touched, even with eyes shut, helps to locate it.

As one might expect, there were far more errors in identifying toes than fingers, and the comments about touch location on the toes may be instructive for SRE of the stroke patient's hand. Several subjects said that the second, third and fourth toes 'feel like one big toe.' Various mental strategies were reported for identifying the middle toes, such as counting ('I count from the big toe or little toe inwards'), or estimating the where-abouts of the touched toe in relation to an imaginary mid-line of the foot. For instance, one subject 'felt the touch not so much on a particular toe, as near or less near to the mid-line of the foot. .. (and) estimated the distance from that line.' Many reported consciously visualizing the foot. With diffi-cult toes 'a definite thought-process went on.' 'You have to see a picture of the foot and fit on the feeling.'

Describing the place touched presents its own problems. One student said 'The finger or toe is identified first: giving it the correct name is a separate operation.' How difficult this 'separate operation' is seems to depend on what response is required. Halnan and Wright list, in order of increasing difficulty: pointing to the spot and touching it (the easiest method), pointing without touching (both of these being easier with

vision than without), pointing to a diagram or model, and – the most difficult – pointing to the examiner's reversed hand.

This illuminating study, though carried out on healthy young adults,
suggests a number of ways for helping a stroke patient learn to discriminate between his fingers. In the first place, the therapist's touch should be
firm ('give a good dig at it'), and the patient should be given plenty of time
to explore the after-effect before moving on to another location.
('Sometimes the tingling remains from the last touch and confuses the
current one. The sensation lasts for quite a long time ...[it] doesn't echo
for so long on the feet as on the hands.') Moving the finger touched clearly
helps to identify it or to confirm an identification already made. Even
having the finger moved by the therapist should help. The patient should
also be encouraged to turn his head towards the part being touched and
then – when he opens his eyes – to gaze at it as he tries to localize the
touch. Subjects' comments reported by Halnan and Wright suggest that
this directing of the gaze may improve tactile localization, and this is
supported by more recent research, mentioned earlier, showing that
reaction time to tactile stimuli decreases if blindfold gaze is directed to the
point stimulated (Honoré, Bourdeaud'hui and Sparrow, 1989; Pierson et
al., 1991). Aid from vision can, in fact, be recruited in a number of ways: by
mentally visualizing the hand, by looking at a picture or model of the
hand, and by directing the gaze to the place touched – both while it is
touched and afterwards.

As in other lessons, it is profitable to begin finger identification with the
good hand, both in order to introduce the subject to the patient and
because improvement in tactile discrimination after practising with one
hand has been shown to transfer to the other hand (Sathian and
Zangaladze, 1997).

The therapist holds the patient's index finger firmly. 'The last finger I
held was the thumb, and you recognized it easily. Try to feel that this one is
near the thumb. Keeping your eyes closed, look at it and then look at the
thumb: look backwards and forwards between the two, keeping your eyes
closed all the time, and try to see that there is no other finger between
them: this must be the index finger. Now I'll move it up and down to help
you feel it.' The same method can be used for focusing on the ring finger if
the patient can identify his little finger. For the third finger: 'It's difficult to
tell the third from the fourth finger, but I'm going to hold the fourth and
fifth together and move the third: try gazing at it and seeing it in the
middle of the hand.'

The third and fourth fingers are the hardest to identify, both for healthy
people and for most stroke patients. The separate identity of these fingers
is so far from most people's consciousness that trying to teach it directly by

touching them is apt with some patients to be an academic and unrewarding task. Such a patient may more easily learn to 'disentangle' these fingers in the course of some of the lessons in proprioception (for instance, Lesson 10) described in the next chapter.

Chapter 8
The curriculum II

Lessons in proprioception

Proprioception, or the sense of one's own body, of its position, configuration and movement from moment to moment, is the most mysterious of all the senses. Its workings seem equally impenetrable to introspection and to scientific study. I can tell, without looking, where my hand or my foot is, but I cannot begin to say how I know this. This most private of all senses did not even figure in Aristotle's list of five senses and only began belatedly to be studied in this century, and our understanding of it is still rudimentary compared with other senses. Excluding the vestibular or balance system of the inner ear which does not concern us here, proprioception is served by receptors in joints, muscles and tendons. In addition, receptors in the skin also contribute information about movement in the joints of the hand (Moberg, 1983; Edin and Abbs, 1991). The proprioceptive system, especially in the hand, is characterized by great redundancy, with many types of receptors signalling information about position and movement with a large degree of overlap. This redundancy presumably makes for greater accuracy, as well as perhaps providing enhanced information about the context and meaning of any sensory signals. It also means that the different receptor systems – in joints, muscle and skin – can to a considerable extent substitute for each other so that, for instance, people who have undergone prosthetic replacement of their metacarpophalangeal joints (the knuckle joints) seem to have unimpaired sensitivity to movement at these artificial joints (Kelso, Holt and Flatt, 1980). Proprioceptors are not only of various kinds but they are also spatially scattered to a remarkable degree. Taking the knuckle joints of the fingers as an example, the movement at these joints that accompanies flexion or extension is signalled by receptors in the joints themselves, by receptors in the overlying skin on the back of the hand and by receptors (muscle spindles) three-quarters of the way up the forearm in the long muscles which flex and extend the fingers.

The fact that the sources of proprioception are so many and so dispersed holds out the possibility, both in peripheral and in central lesions, that some element may persist after injury and serve as the starting off point for sensory re-education. As sense of movement is often less disturbed than sense of position after stroke, we begin the re-education of proprioception with a lesson involving movement.

Lesson 6: Guided drawing

This is an activity that patients enjoy and which can be used for every level of proprioceptive ability. The therapist puts a pencil or marker pen in the patient's hand and, holding the patient's hand in hers, makes a drawing which he has to identify without looking. This makes use of the sense of passive movement to solve a challenging and interesting task.

Since this sensory exercise was developed and described (Yekutiel, 1977), an intriguing study by Roll and Gilhodes has thrown light on the proprioceptive mechanism that enables one to sense what is being drawn with one's passive hand (Roll and Gilhodes, 1995). Vibrating the tendon of a muscle, which excites its muscle spindles (the sensory endings in muscle), gives the subject the illusory sensation that the muscle is being stretched and the joint over which it passes moved – even into a position which is anatomically impossible (Goodwin, McCloskey and Matthews, 1972; Craske, 1977; Lackner, 1988). Roll and Gilhodes vibrated the wrist tendons of nine blindfolded subjects who sat with a pen in their right hand and then asked them to identify the figures which they thought their hand had traced. The tendons were vibrated in sequences and combinations corresponding to the pattern of stretches which would occur in these muscles during the drawing of squares, triangles and other common geometrical shapes. Although they had not in fact drawn anything, the subjects were remarkably confident in their answers: none had any hesitation in stating that they had drawn four-sided or three-sided figures, and there were only a few doubts about the distinction between a square and a rectangle. After decades during which sensory input from muscles was not believed to reach consciousness, this study shows that this information not only is available to consciousness but can evoke quite complex images in the cognitive domain.

The healthy young subjects in these experiments were given no clue as to what figures they were likely to sense. The stroke patient needs to know what possibilities to expect. He is helped to succeed by the use of cards (Fig. 8.1), showing figures which he discusses and names with the therapist and which he looks at while she draws one of them.

Figure 8.1 shows a set of six hand-drawn cards, each with four figures which are progressively harder to distinguish. Card 1 has four variations

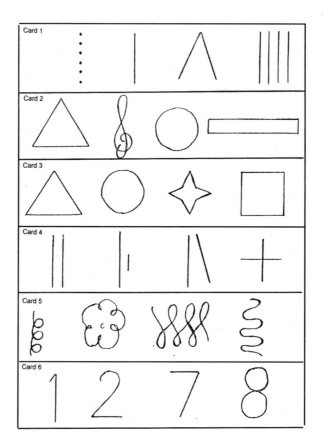

Figure 8.1 Six cards for guided drawing.

on the straight line. Card 2 has four quite dissimilar closed figures, and Card 3 shows closed figures that are harder to distinguish. Card 4 depicts variations on the theme of two lines, while the theme in Card 5 is curves and loops in a constant or a changing direction. Card 6 shows the more easily distinguished numerals, and this can lead on to other numbers, letters, or even whole words and messages. It may surprise the patient to discover that he can recognize 'Good morning! How are you?' when the therapist writes this greeting holding his good hand. Perhaps he can feel some of these letters with his other hand?

As in other lessons, this task is tried out first with the good hand, then with the affected hand while the patient watches, and only then without him seeing his hand. In Figure 8.2 a patient is watching the therapist draw with his affected hand, and Figure 8.3 shows one of many possible arrangements which allows the patient to see the figures but not his hand.

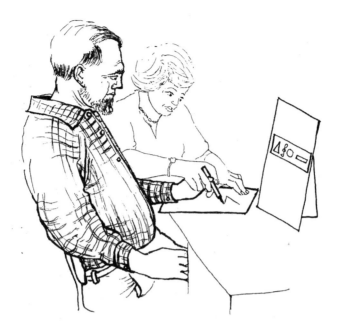

Figure 8.2 Watching guided drawing.

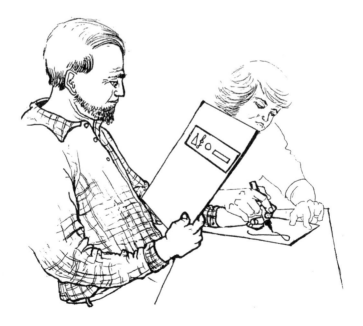

Figure 8.3 Which figure is she drawing?

The preliminary discussion is important. The patient should be encouraged to give names to the figures and identify special features which may help him to recognize them. Looking, for instance, at Card 2 (Fig. 8.1): 'Well, the first is a triangle: I expect I can feel three lines if you separate them clearly enough. The second is a squiggle – no, I know, it's a sign in music. The third is a ball, we'll call it a circle, and the last is a long bar.' He holds the card between himself and the table; the therapist grasps his hand and makes a slow deliberate circle. 'Did you feel any corners? No? Then it must be either the music clef or the circle. I'll do it again. See if it's smooth or a squiggle. If it's the music clef, you may be able to feel that the speed of the pen changes for the loops at the top and bottom' (Schwartz, 1994).

The figures can be drawn very large, with movements of the whole arm, or very small confining the movement to the wrist as in writing. The card can also be turned and stood on its end so that most of the drawing movements are transverse to the body rather than in the sagittal plane, involving what Bernstein (1967) calls 'a quite different muscular formula'. Since a stroke patient's awareness both of his body and of external space may be disturbed in a quite piecemeal fashion (Bisiach, Capitani and Porta, 1985), it is a good idea to carry out the drawings not only in front of the patient but also to his right and to his left side.

Guided drawing involves the sense of movement. The remaining four lessons in proprioception address sense of position.

Lesson 7: Where is your thumb?

The therapist holds the patient's plegic hand in a position which is not painful for him, and he tries without looking to locate it and grasp the thumb with his good hand (Fig. 8.4). It sometimes helps to tie a bright ribbon round the thumb which he has to find. He can also be helped by the therapist making small movements with the hand which she is holding or by himself moving or trying to move it. He should open his eyes the moment he has tried to grasp his thumb.

The therapist needs to be on the look out for variations in the patient's ability to locate his hand in different areas of external space. Many patients are quite accurate when the hand is more or less in front of them, but 'lose it' when it is moved away to one side or above the head. Problematic areas should be identified, discussed and worked at.

Lesson 8: The distance between the hands

It is remarkable how accurately, without looking, one can place one's two hands to indicate the size of an object or even a specified number of inches or centimetres (the angler's exaggerated demonstration of the size

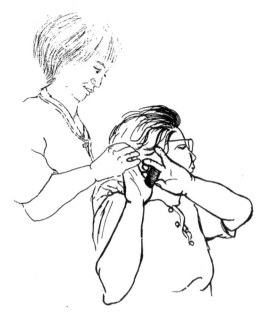

Figure 8.4 Where is your thumb?

of yesterday's catch is caused by wishful thinking rather than faulty proprioception). This feat of proprioception must use information about the width of the shoulders, the length of the arms and forearms and the angular position of shoulders, elbows, forearms and wrists in trigonometric calculations which the owner of the hands may never have mastered – and the feat is achieved instantaneously! It suggests a number of possible SRE exercises in position sense.

With the patient's eyes closed, the therapist places his two palms facing each other at a distance of, say, 2 inches (5 centimetres) and asks 'Do you think you could get your head through the space between your hands? – or a football? – or could I pass my hand through it?'. Alternatively, the therapist can hold the patient's two palms far apart and gradually bring them together, asking him to stop her when he thinks they measure the width of his shoulders, his head, or some object that they have chosen beforehand.

Lesson 9: Identify the position of your hand

The therapist arranges the patient's hand in a certain position – closed or open, fingers together or separated – and asks him to concentrate on trying to feel what position it is in and then to imitate it with his other hand or describe it in words or point to a picture. Figure 8.5 shows eight

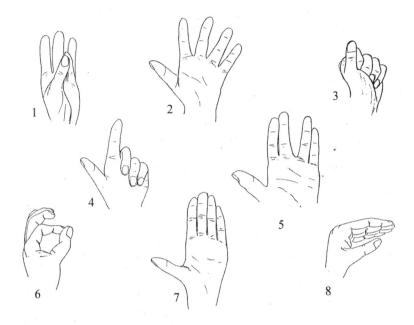

Figure 8.5 Hand positions.

positions of the hand which can be used. Few patients will be able to distinguish all eight, but contrasting positions – like numbers 2 and 3 – can be chosen as a start and other positions gradually added. Painful positions are avoided, but the patient's attention is drawn to feelings of stretch or tightness as well as to whether all or only some of the fingers touch each other, and whether they touch the palm.

Lesson 10: Thick and thin rods

A set of cylindrical wooden rods with diameters ranging from 5 to 30 millimetres can be used for many different lessons with a major proprioceptive component. The patient in Figure 8.6 is trying to decide between which fingers the thickest rod has been placed. This is an advanced lesson. A simpler task is deciding whether it is the thinnest or the thickest that has been placed in the hand or between thumb and index finger or between any pair of fingers. This and the previous lesson on hand position can also be exploited for teaching finger identification.

This lesson with rods already encroaches on the recognition of objects and their qualities, which is the third subject in the curriculum of SRE.

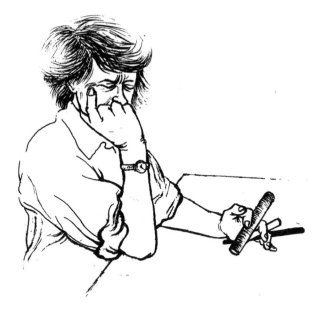

Figure 8.6 Where is the thickest rod?

Lessons in the recognition of objects and their qualities

It takes only a second or two to identify a familiar object held in the hand (Wynn Parry, 1973; Klatzky, Lederman and Metzger, 1985), although we are using input from a large and diverse number of variously located receptors bringing information about different qualities such as shape, size, texture, weight and consistency. We are not normally aware of these different sources of information – sometimes not even of the qualities of the object – which lead to our identifying it: the identification seems to be an immediate and total recognition rather than something built up piecemeal from separate components. And if we are asked afterwards which parts of our hand or which of our fingers touched the object we shall probably be unable to say, although the location of the points of touch and their positions relative to each other must be critical for discerning the object's size and form.

Astereognosis, or the inability to recognize three-dimensional objects by handling them, may be due simply to lack of sensory information, as in peripheral nerve injury, spinal cord lesion or damage to afferent (incoming) nerve tracts at many locations in the brain (Kennedy, 1924). It can also occur, as 'tactile agnosia', when the sensory information is available but the use of this information – the process of selection, integration and interpretation that is presumed to occur – is disturbed. Without entering again into the controversy surrounding tactile agnosia described in Chapter 3, it is clear that astereognosis after stroke is likely to acquire agnostic characteristics even if the primary deficit is sensory. Recall the 'tactile agnosia', described by Leont'ev and Zaporozhets and reviewed in Chapter 4, in patients with severe wounds but with intact central nervous system (Leont'ev and Zaporozhets, 1945/1960).

The lessons in object recognition therefore focus on the acquisition of tactics of perception: that is, on looking for and interpreting the diagnostic clues from whatever sensory information is available. SRE in object recognition involves a lot of discussion of the clues that the patient can use to identify specific objects. The lessons presented here begin with weight, shape and other qualities of objects. It is often easier for a patient to concentrate on one quality – whichever is easiest for him to appreciate – and work at first with objects which differ only in this one quality; he can then go on to other qualities before dealing with a number of qualities. However, this is not always the case: some patients find the lessons in object qualities academic and difficult and should rather start with objects differing widely in a number of qualities. As always, the choice of lessons is dictated by the patient's abilities and by what interests him.

Lesson 11: Weight

Heavy weights held in the hand will be sensed by receptors in the whole limb and even in the trunk and therefore may be the first things that the severely insensate patient can feel. A start can be made by the patient becoming confident and quick at telling the difference between, say, an iron dumb-bell and a light wooden rod (Fig. 8.7) or between a kilo metal disc – such as those used in physiotherapy departments – and a similarly shaped wooden or plastic disc. With the patient's hand resting on the table and, as usual, after experimenting with the good hand, the therapist says 'I'm putting one of these two objects on your hand. If it's the heavy one, you'll feel it pressing on your hand even before you try to lift it. You think it's the heavy one? Well, just to confirm this, try to lift it. If it's the heavy one, you will feel the weight all the way up your arm. Yes, of course, you were right. Look, it's the dumb-bell.'

All sorts of similarly shaped objects of different weight can be used for teaching weight discrimination, but the subject is not interesting enough to merit more than a small part of the time available for SRE. Like the early lessons in touch (lessons 1 and 2), weight discrimination is valuable chiefly as a way to show the patient that his hand is not as useless as he thought, that there is at least one quality of objects that he can sense.

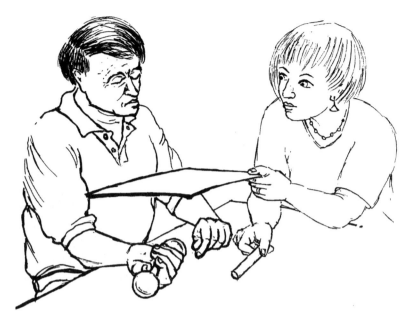

Figure 8.7 Weight discrimination.

Lesson 12: Shape – the Pellenberg Box

According to the very thorough investigation that Lederman and Klatzky made of the recognition of common objects by the hand, shape is by far the most frequent 'main diagnostic attribute' (Lederman and Klatzky, 1990). Shape discrimination is therefore a key subject in the re-education of object recognition. It is a special aspect of the ability to deal with spatial relations (Semmes, 1965) and can be selectively impaired in stroke patients, with other sensory functions left intact (Reed, Caselli and Farah, 1996). It should be taught through direct work on shapes and emphasized when working with objects differing in many qualities.

Of the many ways of teaching shape discrimination the best is perhaps by the Pellenberg box. This was the brainchild of Heidi Lemmens, a therapist working at the Pellenberg Rehabilitation Centre in Leuven in Belgium, who designed the box after hearing about SRE. A modification of the Pellenberg box and some of its contents is shown in Figure 8.8, and a patient can be seen using it in Figure 8.9. The box contains some twenty pairs of wooden shapes, with one of each pair mounted on a square piece of plywood which can be placed on the lid of the box and the other left unmounted. The original Pellenberg box had only the mounted shapes, which the patient traced with his fingers – or was helped to trace – while

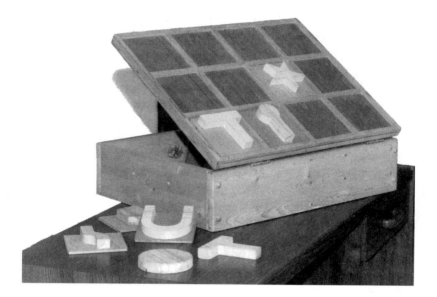

Figure 8.8 The Pellenberg box.

his arm rested on a padded roller-skate (Fig. 7.4, p 82). This seems to place too much constraint on the patient's tactics of perception. 'Following the contour' is indeed one of the two exploratory procedures used for judging the shape of an object – the other is 'enclosure' (Lederman and Klatzky, 1990) – but the common objects of everyday life that the hand normally recognizes so quickly have three-dimensional contours, and we are poor at recognizing two-dimensional patterns with our fingers (Klatzky and Lederman, 1987; Reed, 1994). The addition of unmounted copies of the shapes creates a larger repertoire of exercises using varied tactics of perception. At the simplest level, the patient can identify the special features of one of the free objects with his good hand – the points of the star or the smooth continuity of the circle – and then try to find these features when the object is 'manipulated' in his plegic hand. He can handle a free shape while looking at shapes mounted on the lid of the box. He can trace a mounted shape with one hand while handling its twin with the other hand (Figure 8.9), and the two hands can exchange roles.

All these exercises are preceded by the patient choosing and naming the shapes that he thinks he may be able to recognize. The importance of the patient giving names to the objects or figures on which he is going to concentrate has been mentioned already in a number of contexts. The time has come to justify this, even if this can be done only by citing authorities who bear only obliquely on the issue. William James, who devoted

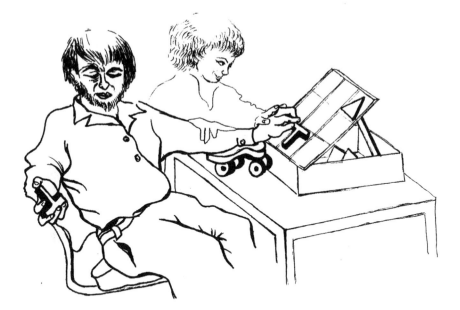

Figure 8.9 Using the Pellenberg box.

one of the longest chapters in his 'Principles of Psychology' to the subject of 'Discrimination and Comparison', rather surprisingly did not directly address the importance of naming in our perception of things, but it is implicit in many passages. A good example is his discussion of 'how does one learn to distinguish claret from burgundy?' (James, 1890). Through repeated experience, 'the adhesion of each wine with its own *name* [James' italics] becomes more and more inveterate, and at last each flavour suggests instantly and certainly its own name and nothing else. The names differ far more than the flavours, and help to stretch these latter farther apart.' James stresses the differentiating role of names. Gibson also stressed the contribution of language to the development of perception in childhood: 'talking fixes the gains of perceiving' (Gibson, 1966). Most relevant is the work of Marr, whose model of information-processing underlying visual object recognition had widespread influence in cognitive psychology (Marr, 1976). Marr enunciated what he called 'the principle of explicit naming' which, loosely translated for our purpose, refers to the economy and efficiency that the use of names (or symbols) can be expected to contribute to the processing, retrieving and general handling of information. It therefore seems likely that the act of giving a name to an object or figure helps to direct the patient's attention to it and fix it in his memory as one of the objects he is going to feel with his hand.

On a more practical level, it is clearly important for the therapist and patient to establish a common language. If the patient decides to call the circular Pellenberg shape a 'biscuit' or a 'cookie', this should be clear at the outset so that the therapist does not think that he is referring to any number of other biscuit-like shapes! It is also important to be sure that he distinguishes the shapes visually – that, for instance, he does not call all quadrilateral figures 'squares' or 'boxes' or whatever. People vary considerably in the size and use of their vocabulary, and they do not become more articulate after a stroke. The therapist will often have to help the patient find names for the objects he is going to study, and this is part of the discussion that launches a new sensory task .

Lesson 13: Coloured bricks

This is another lesson in shape discrimination, which uses more easily obtainable objects than the Pellenberg box. All that is needed is a selection of identical pairs of children's coloured bricks. Figure 8.10 shows a patient looking at a number of bricks and deliberating which of them is the twin of the one in his hand. The matching of paired objects in this and the previous lesson is particularly suitable for severely aphasic patients.

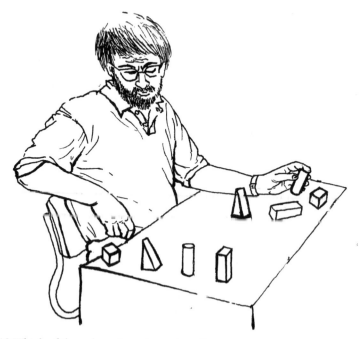

Figure 8.10 Which of these have I got in my hand?

Lesson 14: Size

The perception of the size of an object held in the hand is a predominantly proprioceptive function in that knowledge of the object's dimensions must come from information about the position and configuration of the hand and fingers. It was pointed out earlier that proprioception is an inseparable element in the hand's perceptual (haptic) functions and that the classically distinguished exteroceptive and proprioceptive systems are closely interwoven in everyday life. The subject divisions in the curriculum are correspondingly blurred, and a start was already made – under 'Proprioception' – towards teaching size discrimination using rods of different diameters (Lesson 10).

The round lids of jars of different sizes provide a useful way for teaching size discrimination. Even a patient with very reduced sensation can usually tell when his fingers are spread and know, therefore, that he's holding a large rather than a small lid (Fig. 8.11). Other possibilities are smooth pebbles of various sizes, pencils of different lengths, balls of different sizes, children's wooden bricks of different dimensions, and the set of rods already used.

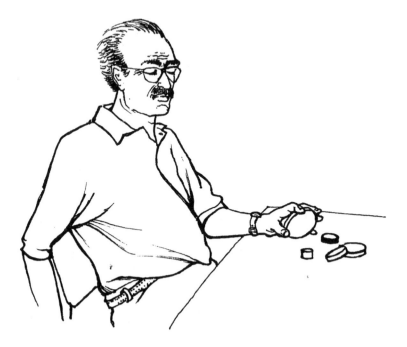

Figure 8.11 Size discrimination.

Lesson 15: Consistency

Consistency – or hardness – is another diagnostic attribute used, only slightly less frequently than weight, for recognizing objects (Lederman and Klatzky, 1990). It is judged by pressing or squeezing the object, even the slightest pressure often being enough to show whether it is hard or soft and deformable. For studying this, objects are chosen whose main difference is their 'squeezability', such as solid and hollow rubber tubes, a ball of knitting wool and a tennis ball.

Lesson 16: Temperature

Temperature is often a useful clue, for instance for distinguishing between metal and wood, and perception of temperature tends to be relatively preserved after stroke. The temperature of an object held in the hand can also be judged without having to lift it or manipulate it. However, it is not sufficiently interesting to be taught as a separate subject. Temperature should be noted as a possible clue for object recognition and the patient's attention drawn to it when relevant.

Lesson 17: Texture

Texture discrimination has already been presented in Lesson 4 as part of the curriculum for touch. It can also be taught as an important diagnostic quality – ranking almost equal to size – for identifying objects. The patient in Figure 8.12 is trying to decide whether she has the rough or the smooth stone in her hand. Other pairs of objects for this sort of lesson are a fir cone and an apple, ropes and rubber tubes, and coasters made of plastic or glass or various fibres.

Lesson 18: Object recognition

We noted earlier that our hands normally recognize common objects so rapidly that, as with so many everyday feats of perception, we often cannot say immediately how this recognition came about. Even if the underlying neurophysiological processes are completely inaccessible to introspection, a little thought and a few repetitions of the act are usually sufficient at least to identify what Lederman and Klatzky (1990) called the 'diagnostic attributes' of the object and the 'exploratory procedures' which the hand used to search for and find these attributes. Both the diagnostic attributes and the exploratory procedures need to be studied and discussed thoroughly with the patient before making any attempts with the affected hand. The therapist asks him to choose from a variety of objects spread out on the table in front of him two or more that he thinks he may be able to tell apart with his affected hand, to name them and to point out the features that he will look

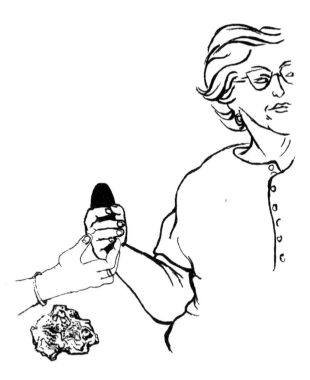

Figure 8.12 The rough or the smooth stone?

for. If, for instance, he chooses a fir cone and a short iron pipe, there will be many clues – from shape, weight, consistency, texture and temperature. He closes his eyes, and the therapist puts the fir cone in his good hand. 'Well, this is the fir cone – I can tell at once'. 'Good. Now check one by one for each of the clues you said would help, and try to feel what you do with your hand to find each clue.' This should be done very slowly with the fir cone and then with the iron pipe. The patient can open his eyes from time to time to see what he does with his hand as he checks for the different clues. The therapist also observes these exploratory procedures very carefully, because she may have to help him use them when he works with his affected hand. If the patient has little voluntary hand movement she must try to reproduce the procedures as she moves his hand over the object or moves the object in his hand, all the time describing what she is doing. If he has some ability to hold the object and manipulate it, her contribution will be to remind him what he did with his good hand: 'What did you do with your other hand to judge the thing's weight? Yes, you lifted it', or 'Didn't you rub your thumb along it to see whether it's rough or smooth?' The patient can profitably open his eyes from time to time. Remember that this is not an examination or a competition!

When the patient has become accurate and confident at recognizing objects when there are only two alternatives and these are two objects which he himself has chosen, the moment has come to increase the number of objects by combining pairs which he has worked with, so that he now has to discriminate between four or more objects, all of which he has seen and handled recently (Fig. 8.13). This is rather like the common everyday action of getting something out of a drawer or a handbag without looking. The possibilities are limited, and one needs very few clues to pick the desired object. Feeling for a pen or pencil in one's handbag, one doesn't need to check the ends to be sure it isn't a toothbrush!

The next stage of difficulty opens the field to unknown objects. The therapist warns the patient that she is going to add a new object to the two (or more) which he already recognizes. If he cannot identify it but is sure that it is neither the fir cone nor the iron pipe he can just call it 'the unknown', but perhaps he can hazard a guess as to what it is. She gives him a folded pair of socks: 'Yes, you're right, this is the unknown. What can you say about it? Is it heavy? Can you squeeze it? Is it hard or soft? What could it be?'

To narrow the number of possibilities, the therapist and patient can decide that all the objects she will give him are work tools or things to be found on a desk or in a bathroom, and he can be helped beforehand by

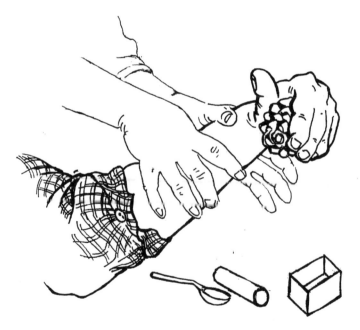

Figure 8.13 'This is the fir cone'.

naming the objects she might hand him. Whenever a new type of exercise shows signs of being beyond the patient's abilities, he should immediately return to a task which he can do.

There are endless ways for practising object recognition, and the therapist should look beyond her desk and kitchen drawer for possible objects. Children's small wooden or plastic animals, leaves and stones all add to the interest of SRE. Probably the least fruitful method is to present an arbitrary series of objects, as this sort of open-ended exercise may seem to the patient to have neither a goal nor a conclusion. It is better to structure the task and agree on it explicitly with the patient, for instance by asking him to choose a number of objects which have something in common. The therapist can also ask him how many of the objects which he has already distinguished when they were presented in pairs he thinks he can recognize when she chooses from the whole set. This gives him a clear goal and a challenge: namely, to get 5 out of 5 or 10 out of 10.

Suggestions for homework

If motivation and interest are the cardinal ingredients for successful sensory re-education of the hand after stroke, third in order of importance is time spent on practice. Even if it is possible for the patient to have daily sessions with the therapist or to follow Wynn Parry's prescription of four ten-minute sessions every day (Wynn Parry and Salter, 1976), he should be encouraged to practise by himself as much as possible. Independent practice will help to consolidate what he has learned and to link his improving sensation to daily life activities. It also serves to acknowledge and endorse his active role in his own rehabilitation.

There are patients who find SRE so encouraging and so fascinating that they are eager to practise on their own. These patients can be a rich source of ideas for new methods of sensory re-education. On the other hand, given the fact that stroke patients tend to suffer from feelings of depression and helplessness, many will be less compliant and will not easily be persuaded to do something for themselves in the form of independent and often unaided homework. General advice to practise is not likely to be effective. As with other aspects of SRE, the therapist and the patient need to discuss the question of homework together and arrive at decisions that are both mutually agreed on and specific as to 'what', 'when' and 'how'. If possible, the co-operation of relatives or other regular visitors should be enlisted.

Some form of self-monitoring such as a diary is useful. At the end of each session, the therapist gives the patient whatever equipment he will need for his homework, and she or the patient notes in the diary the tasks and the times at which he has decided to do them. The patient then ticks them off as he does them. In general, the greater the patient's involvement in all the decisions about homework, and the more specific and structured the assignment, the greater the likelihood that he will succeed in carrying it out. If he does not manage to do the homework – and the system 'doesn't work' – it must be changed until success, however small, is achieved. Whatever homework is chosen, the patient and therapist should run through it before the session ends. The following are suggestions for homework that patients can do between sessions.

1. **Where is my thumb?** The patient closes his eyes and tries to grasp his plegic thumb with his good hand. If he misses, he looks to see in what direction he erred. He can do this at prescribed times or at any moment in the day – when he wakes from a nap or when, as is the case for so much of the day, he is just sitting doing nothing.
2. **What is my hand doing?** The patient tries to feel not only where his hand is but also what position it is in. Are the fingers open or closed, and what is each finger touching? He can do this when he is sitting or lying down. He can also try to gauge the angle of his elbow.
3. **Buttons** Many of the two-handed exercises with buttons used by occupational therapists can be profitably practised with eyes shut, the two hands taking it in turns to hold the button or the cloth. The patient can also find and count the buttons on his shirt.
4. **What is in the bag?** The patient takes away from the session a cloth bag containing a number of objects (not too many) which he has already identified successfully with his hand. After experimenting with his good hand, he puts his plegic hand into the bag – with help from his other hand if necessary – and either identifies the objects as he finds them or decides that he is going to look for a specific object This replicates a fairly common everyday activity. The patient should choose different objects after each session: fewer and easier ones if he got discouraged, different ones if he found it easy.
5. **Blindfold drawing** If the patient has better powers of movement than sensation, he may be able to hold a fat felt-tip pen or marker and draw or write. He can set himself, with eyes shut, to draw a circle or a square or write a number or a letter or even a word, and he can practise this alternately with his good hand and with his affected hand. He will find that the performance of both hands improves rapidly with practice.

The choice of homework has to take into account the practical question of what the patient can do alone and what help he has from his family. Within these limits, however, it is guided by the same general principles that govern SRE. The tasks must be interesting if they are to engage the patient's attention rather than being repeated mechanically. They should be within the patient's powers but difficult enough to present some challenge. They should include aspects of the three subjects of the curriculum – touch, proprioception and object recognition – in whatever proportion seems appropriate for the individual patient. Finally, when rehearsing the homework at the end of the session, the therapist should be sure that the patient uses his main tools for SRE, namely his mind, his eyes and his good hand. He should decide before each task what he is going to do and name the object or the task to himself. He should practise it first with his good hand, and he should check himself throughout by opening his eyes and looking.

Both the patient and the therapist will find that they tend to choose too much homework. The therapist's ambition, together with the heightened confidence of the patient at the end of the session, make this tendency almost irresistible, but it is wise to decide on too little rather than too much. The tasks should also err towards being too easy. It is vital to avoid failure and discouragement. The purpose of the homework is practice, or the repetition and perfecting of what the patient has already learned to do.

Chapter 9
Validation of the method

In Chapter 2 we looked at the present state of therapy for stroke patients and saw that the results of trials to evaluate its effectiveness have been inconclusive. Current therapy is, in fact, based on concepts and methods that still await validation.

There are historical reasons for this state of affairs. The most commonly used therapies for stroke patients today, namely those associated with the names of Brunnstrom and Bobath, were developed in the 1950s and 1960s. They were based on clinical experience, with some theoretical rationale drawn from what was then the classical neurophysiology of Hughlings Jackson, Magnus and Sherrington. Although it was in those decades that the medical profession accepted the idea of a controlled clinical trial as a prerequisite for the use of drugs and vaccines, non-pharmacological therapy was not – and to a great extent still is not – expected to submit to scientific evaluation. Innovators of therapeutic methods are, in general, the last people to feel that an unbiased evaluation of their methods is necessary. As Bach-y-Rita pointed out, 'the very person-ality traits that make these practitioners successful with patients (supreme, unquestioning confidence) make them poor candidates to carry out a scientific study' (Bach-y-Rita, 1986). The priority for them is to spread the word. 'These often charismatic leaders peddled belief systems, demanded obedience, taught complex and difficult treatment regimes and provided a reward system which ensured the continued maintenance of their own clinical approach to specific problems' (Twomey, 1996). Their methods for treating stroke patients were disseminated throughout the profession at a time when the validation of therapeutic methods by clinical trials was not yet de rigueur. By the time some evidence of therapeutic efficacy began to be demanded, it had become unthinkable to deprive stroke patients of this accepted therapy, and the few clinical trials that were carried out consisted for the most part of comparisons between different types of therapy, rather than between therapy and no therapy. The results of these trials showed no clear advantage for any one method, leaving it in doubt whether all are efficacious, or none of them. As Partridge and de Weerdt have pointed out, 'though the theoretical and practical differences between the various named approaches to physiotherapy for stroke are often stressed by their proponents, scrutiny of the original concepts shows that they actually have much in common. This may be one reason why comparative studies have failed to find significant differences in the results achieved' (Partridge and de Weerdt, 1995). At best, the prevention of contractures in conjunction with the well-meaning attention and encouragement to move that are common to therapy in every school of thought may represent a regime – with a large placebo component – that is helpful after stroke. At worst, the functional outcome for the patient is not affected by any of the methods advocated. Recall that the study of patients receiving minimal or no rehabil- itation in Soweto in South Africa found that these patients, discharged from hospital an average of ten days after stroke, reached a standard of indepen- dent walking comparable to that achieved by stroke patients in the West after lengthy in-patient rehabilitation (Hale and Eales, 1998).

Today, in the case of a therapeutic approach believed to be new, there is no justification for encouraging it to be practised widely before its effect has been properly assessed. This was the train of thought that led to the decision to carry out a trial of SRE before promoting its wider use in stroke rehabilitation.

Theoretical considerations

It must be stated, in defence of the generations of therapists who have with great dedication used unproved methods of treatment, that the task of evaluating the effect of a specific therapy on the recovery of stroke patients is beset by enormous difficulties. These difficulties go far beyond the natural reluctance of therapists to use precious work time for taking a critical look at their practice: they are intrinsic to the subject. They arise primarily from the problem of separating the effects of therapy from those of spontaneous recovery.

It is clear that whatever processes of neuroplasticity are set in train after stroke, these will be at their maximum during the first few weeks or months. This follows from the neurophysiological literature and is borne out by the data on the time course of recovery of patients, whether expressed in terms of impairment or in terms of disability (Kelly-Hayes et al., 1989). The first months are therefore the time to provide the patient with every sort of therapy likely to enhance his recovery. However, this is a very problematic period for research on therapeutic efficacy since it is diffi- cult to separate the effects of intervention from those of spontaneous recovery. This would not be so difficult if it were possible to predict the amount of recovery likely to occur in individual patients. But in spite of a large amount of research on the prediction of outcome after stroke, there is considerable disagreement about the relative weight of different predicting factors, and the correlations between predictors and outcome measures tend to be low and to have large standard errors (Wade, Wood and Langton Hewer, 1985). The extent and pattern of recovery after stroke vary enormously from patient to patient. Some spontaneous recovery occurs in the vast majority of patients after stroke, and part of the improvement credited to therapy – but no one knows how much – should undoubtedly be attributed to this spontaneous recovery (Kwakkel, Kollen and Wagenaar, 1999). It is clear that any trial of therapy during the period of spontaneous recovery must compare outcome in patients who received the therapy with outcome in patients who did not receive it: this control group of patients is necessary to show what happens when the therapy is not given.

Another confounding factor during the period of rehabilitation is medication. Medical treatment, given according to the patients' individual needs, varies both from patient to patient and from stage to stage for any one patient. This is just one aspect, though perhaps the most important one, of the fact that the patients in whom the effect of one specific therapy is being studied are at the same time receiving a whole arsenal of other medical and non-medical treatments.

In summary, the problem of evaluating the effect of a specific therapy used during the early period of rehabilitation after stroke is that of disentangling it from the effects of a large number of other variables. First and foremost among these variables is the degree of spontaneous recovery of function, itself related not only to pathological and clinical characteristics of the stroke, but also to a complex of positive and negative personal factors which each patient brings to his convalescence and whose influence is imponderable. The second group of variables are those related to other interventions. During the dynamic and life-threatening period of rehabilitation after stroke, the patient is given the benefit of all that the multi-disciplinary team can offer, and by the nature of things this can change from day to day In fact, the period of in-hospital rehabilitation generally continues as long as the patient's functional condition is improving, and stops when it has reached a 'plateau'.

A sobering note about the problem posed to researchers by the enormous variability inherent in patients' situation after stroke is sounded by a recent calculation that a controlled trial to measure the effect of any one of the various neuroprotective agents presently available should include 'several tens of thousands of patients' in order to detect 'moderate clinical benefits' (Dorman and Sandercock, 1996).

One way of avoiding the problem of disentangling the effects of therapy from those of spontaneous recovery and other ongoing interventions is to give the therapy after the period of rehabilitation. When the patient's status has stopped improving and has reached a steady state or 'plateau', any change occurring after a new intervention will be discernible – will, as it were, stand out. Therapy is presumably less likely to change the status of the patient in this chronic phase, but if it is effective in these patients it should be even more effective when given during the dynamic recovery period after stroke. This reasoning dictated the choice of patients one year or more after stroke for a study of the effects of gait training (Wade et al., 1992), for a study of training in a motor task (Dean and Shepherd, 1997) and for the trial of SRE which will now be described.

A controlled trial

The trial of SRE was carried out in patients two or more years after stroke. This left a safe margin of time beyond the period of spontaneous recovery. Although a full report of the trial has been published (Yekutiel and Guttman, 1993), the validity of SRE is such an important part of the presentation of the method that a full description of the basis for this validity is given here, with the added incentive of being able to include details, nuances and thoughts which had no place in the original report.

The patients

Twenty patients were recruited from lists of chronic hemiplegic patients provided by primary health care clinics of the Israel health insurance funds. The main criterion for admission to the trial was the existence of persistent sensory deficit in the hand two or more years after a major stroke. This was established by standard neurological examinations of sense of touch, sense of position and recognition of everyday objects placed in the hand. Patients also had to be over the age of 40 and have no communication problem or significant cognitive or emotional disturbance. They gave informed consent.

Since the study had at the outset been designed to rule out the possibility of spontaneous improvement, it was not at first deemed necessary to include an untreated control group. However, patients were to be assessed with the same battery of sensory tests before and after exposure to SRE, and it was theoretically possible that they would perform better on tests the second time round without there having been any actual improvement in sensory function. A number of authorities have mentioned their impression that sensory test results – notably for two-point discrimination – improve with repetition (James, 1890; Head, 1918).

To control for a possible learning effect of repeating the sensory tests, a second group of 20 patients was recruited from the same source and according to the same criteria. Mean age was slightly but not significantly higher in this group than in the group to be treated (67 years compared with 64). Both groups comprised equal numbers of patients with left and right hemisphere stroke, with the time since stroke ranging from 2 to 18 years (mean of 6.2 years in both groups). Although the allocation to treatment and no treatment was not random, the two groups were highly comparable.

All patients were tested in their homes (by myself) before and after a period of six weeks during which control patients were not seen, while the treated patients had individual lessons of 45 minutes in their homes (from my colleague, Evelyn Guttman) three times a week for six weeks. These lessons followed the principles and methods of SRE that have been described in previous chapters.

The outcome measures

The choice of outcome measures is a critical element in designing therapeutic trials, and – as pointed out in a review of research on physiotherapy for stroke patients – 'key outcome measures have not always been appropriately linked with physiotherapy aims' (Ashburn, Partridge and De Souza, 1993). Our study aimed to find out whether SRE could alleviate severe and long-standing loss of sensory function in the hands of patients after stroke. This was seen as comparable, in the area of motor function, to the much needed investigation of whether present methods of physiotherapy are able to reduce spasticity. Reduction in either sensory deficit or spasticity may be expected to have a beneficial effect on patients' functional abilities in daily life, but it seems logical to establish conclusively that therapy reduces the impairment before exploring the effects that this reduction may have on disability. As Bradford Hill, one of the founders of the concept of the clinical trial, wrote: 'Too often an attempt to answer many questions at one time results in answering none wholly or none clearly' (Hill, 1962). This trial was therefore limited to assessing the effect of SRE on the sensory function of the hand. No attempt was made to encourage patients to use the hand more in their daily lives. Sensation in the hand was both the sole target of the intervention and the outcome assessed by the testing procedure.

Sensory testing was carried out according to a detailed protocol, including the exact words to be used and the technique and duration of stimuli. Testing was done slowly, with pauses between stimuli and several periods of rest. Patients were never told whether their answers were right or wrong, and none of the test tasks or objects was ever used in the sessions of sensory re-education. There were four groups of tests:

1) Location of touch. The patient's hand was inserted under a curtain covering the near side of a small stool on which stood a sketch of the right or left hand divided into 16 areas. This can be seen in Figure 9.1. After ensuring that the patient understood the test by his being able to answer or indicate the correct numbers for touches on the thumb and little finger of his good hand, he was tested with 20 touches on his affected hand. Touch, with a blunt pencil, was made firmly, causing a slight indentation and blanching with a radius of about 2 mm, and maintained for two seconds. Half scores were given for identifying the right finger but not the phalanx, or for identifying the palm but not the area.
2) Sense of elbow position. Blindfolded, the patient was asked to match with his good arm a series of 10 elbow positions of his affected arm. The angle of both elbows was measured with a standard goniometer.

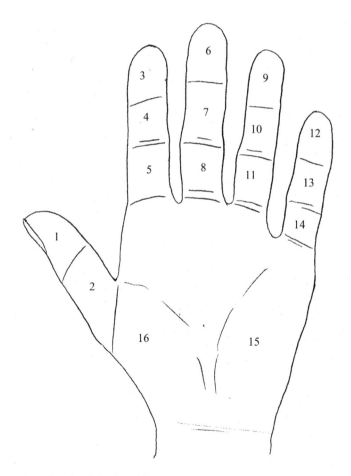

Figure 9.1 Sketch of the hand for testing localization of touch.

3) Two-point discrimination. This was tested on fingers, palm and forearm using a wooden octagon mounted with pins, with pairs of pin-heads separated by 1–5 cms (Fig. 9.2). No attempt was made to establish a two-point threshold, but the patient was asked to state whether he felt one or two points; 32 locations were tested, 9 of them with one point.

4) Tactile object recognition. A tray with 30 everyday objects not used in sensory training – such as a pair of spectacles, a plastic cup, a duster – was shown to the patient in order to find out what name or language he would use. He was then blindfolded and asked to identify a fixed series of 20 of these objects placed in his hand. For those with poor motor function, the examiner moved the object in the patient's hand. The maximum time allowed was 15 seconds. Partial scores were given for recognizing attributes of the object ('heavy', 'plastic', etc.) without identifying it.

Scores on all tests were expressed as percentages.

The results and their interpretation

The treatment and control groups had very similar scores on sensory tests at the outset of the trial, with an average score for the four tests of 43.6% for the control group and 41.7% for the group to be treated. At the second examination six weeks later the control group's scores showed negligible

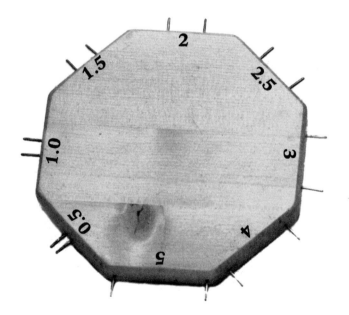

Figure 9.2 Wooden octagon for testing two-point discrimination.

changes, ranging from −1 to +1.4, and an average score of 44.1%. Mean scores of the treated patients, by contrast, showed large increases, all of them statistically significant (P< 0.001), and the average score had risen to 61.7 (P<0.0001). The results are shown in the table below and illustrated in Figure 9.3.

Table 9.1 Percentage scores of 20 treated patients on sensory tests before and after treatment: mean (SE)

Test	Before	After	P*
1 Location of touch	33.7	55.1	0.001
	(5.39)	(5.32)	
2 Sense of elbow position	77.2	85.4	0.001
	(2.38)	(1.48)	
3 Two-point discrimination	25.8	48.1	0.001
	(4.61)	(3.73)	
4 Stereognosis	29.5	56.8	0.0001
	(4.58)	(4.85)	
Total score	41.7	61.7	0.0001
	(2.80)	(3.22)	

*These are two-tailed levels of statistical significance from t tests on the difference between the means of paired samples

(From the Journal of Neurology, Neurosurgery, and Psychiatry 1993 56: 241–244, with permission from the BMJ Publishing Group)

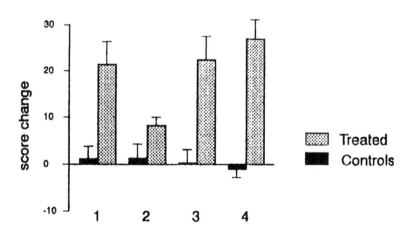

Figure 9.3 Change in percentage scores on tests 1-4: means and standard errors.

The high levels of statistical significance of the changes in sensory scores that occurred after treatment are derived from t-tests on the means of paired samples. This parametric test is not seriously affected by non-normality (Lapin, 1975), but we took two precautions in order to make doubly sure: we normalized the raw data and recalculated the t values, and we used the non-parametric Sign test. Both produced a slight reduction in the statistical significance of the differences between scores before and after treatment, but none fell below the 0.01 level.

Before concluding that the therapeutic effect of SRE has been established and the method validated, two possible flaws in the methodology must be considered. The first is the non-random allocation of patients to the treatment or no treatment groups. Although a randomly assigned control group has come to be seen as an integral part of the design of the clinical trial, neither a control group nor random allocation is always necessary. In a stable situation, where spontaneous improvement is highly unlikely, there is little need to measure what would have happened without the intervention. Bradford Hill cites the hypothetical case of evaluating a new treatment for a disease with 100% mortality (Hill, 1962), but an intervention aimed at chronic impairment in patients years after stroke can serve equally well. The only change likely to occur in an untreated group of such patients is in the direction of deterioration (Wade et al., 1992). As already described, the control patients were recruited in order to check, not for the possibility of spontaneous improvement, but for any learning effect of repeating the sensory tests. The absence of change in their sensory scores rules out the possibility that the higher scores of the treated patients at their second testing could have resulted from their learning how to do the tests.

Although not allocated randomly, the treated and untreated patients were recruited from the same source and according to the same criteria; they showed no differences approaching statistical significance in their distribution by age, duration or laterality of stroke or in their sensory scores at outset. If it is deemed necessary to show that the sensory function of the hand does not improve spontaneously two or more years after stroke, the absence of change in this untreated group confirms this. In fact, Pearson coefficients of correlation between their two sets of scores can be used to measure the test-retest reliability of the tests: they give a reliability of 95% for the total score and a range of 83% to 97% for the four component tests.

The second methodological issue to be considered is the possibility of observer bias, since the examiner was in many cases not blind to the patient's allocation. We attempted to reduce the possible effects of bias to a minimum by using a very precise protocol which prevented any variation in the way the tests were administered, as well as by recording the exact responses of the patient and by using a predetermined and objective system for scoring the answers. The mere possibility of bias, however, remains a serious flaw – so serious that, if the improvement in the patients' sensory scores had been smaller and merely statistically significant, we might have refrained from publishing. As it is, both the precautions taken and the sheer magnitude of the difference of the outcome in the two groups make it unlikely that the results were seriously affected by bias.

Up to now we have been looking at group averages which, with the two caveats just discussed, provide the validation of SRE that was sought. Group averages, however, tend to conceal individual variation which, though treated by the statistician as 'error', can tell us a lot about the response of individual patients. In the present case, individual response to SRE ranged from a gain of one point out of 100 to a gain of 54, in other words from total failure to dramatic success. This suggests either that sensory loss is in some cases irremediable or that the approach used was not appropriate in every case for the specific sensory disturbance. We searched for factors that might differentiate the patients who responded to SRE from those who did not. The two most obvious variables, both of which had a large range – age (from 44-81 years) and time since stroke (2-18 years) – showed no correlation with gains on sensory tests after treatment. The women patients had larger gains than the men (22.6 compared with 18.5), but the difference is neither clinically nor statistically significant. There was a significant inverse correlation between gain and sensory score at outset, patients with greater sensory deficit gaining more than those with less deficit, but this is a statistical artifact (Huskisson, 1974). The only meaningful association found was with the side of the brain damage: on all tests patients with right hemisphere stroke (RHS) showed poorer gains than patients with left hemisphere stroke (LHS), although their sensory scores before treatment were similar. The difference was particularly marked for the tests of two-point discrimination and object recognition in which the gains of the RHS patients, though statistically significant, were less than half of those of the LHS patients. This suggests, to quote from our report of the trial, that 'the method used – although aimed at higher brain centres – may still be too 'peripheral' ... [and] it is possible that the somatosensory deficit in some of the RHS patients was part of a wider perceptual disturbance or hemi-neglect which was neither explored nor addressed in this study' (Yekutiel and Guttman, 1993). The RHS patients may have had a specially impaired ability to deal with spatial relations (Head, 1918; Semmes, 1965).

The next step

The 64-dollar question, and one that was put to me as soon as the study was published – by Dr. Wynn Parry, by the late Dr. Eric Moberg, and by many others – is: what effect does SRE have on the patient's motor function and on his disability in everyday life? As we rigorously avoided 'contaminating' our sensory study by any effort to influence patients' daily life behaviour and made no attempt to evaluate it, we in effect avoided the question. Our star pupil, a 63-year-old woman seven years after major left hemisphere stroke whose average gain of 54 points was the highest, remarked that she could now find things in her kitchen drawer without looking, and another patient also said that he found he could use his hand much more than before. These were unsolicited comments. Our general impression, which was not an encouraging start to the study, was that we were dealing in the main with a group of chronic invalids who had long ago become dependent on assistance from relatives and social services and had neither hope nor motivation for change. If their daily habits were to be changed to exploit their improved hand sensation, it would require very intensive training of a type quite different from SRE. However, my correspondents had raised a very important question.

There are other unanswered questions, the first being whether our research findings are applicable to acute stroke patients. Implicit in the decision to conduct the SRE trial, for methodological reasons, in patients after the period of spontaneous recovery was the idea that if it were effective in chronic patients it should surely be as effective – perhaps even more effective – in the dynamic recovery period immediately after stroke. This is a logical supposition, but it still has to be tested.

There also seems to be a need to develop and evaluate special methods of SRE for some patients with right hemisphere stroke whose sensory deficit may be part of – or accompanied by – various types of agnosia and neglect.

Another question that the study raises is: what actually happened in the brain of a patient like our star pupil, who at outset felt nothing when objects were put in her hand but six weeks later was aware of all 20 objects and correctly named 15 of them? The review in Chapter 4 suggests that there are many different ways in which brain function can change in response to demand, whether posed by learning or by stroke or other injury, and therefore an equivalent number of models or hypotheses that can be proposed to explain improvement in sensory function after SRE. Although the answer must await progress in our understanding of the neurophysiological basis of recovery and learning, much could already be learned by carrying out some form of monitoring of the brain's handling of sensory input in patients receiving SRE. It could be illuminating, for instance, to compare the sensory evoked potentials (SEPs) – the record of

the brain's reception and transmission of sensory input from the hand –
before and after SRE in patients whose hand sensation improved and in
patients who did not improve.

Taken together, these questions point towards two directions for future
work. The first is to tackle the thorny problem of trying to assess the effects
of SRE on both sensory and motor function in various types of patients
during rehabilitation, possibly with the aid of sensory evoked potentials or
other non-invasive techniques for observing brain function. In view of the
methodological difficulties inherent in therapeutic trials during stroke
rehabilitation, the subject should probably be approached by means of in-
depth case studies.

The second direction for future work is towards integrating the principles of SRE into the overall regime of stroke rehabilitation. All members
of the rehabilitation team should at the least be aware of the patient's
sensory problems and be kept informed about any change that occurs so
that they can, on the one hand, adjust their treatment to the existence of
sensory loss and, on the other hand, exploit and build on whatever
sensory improvement occurs. For instance, patients should work at
improving their manual dexterity and their sensory discrimination at the
same time. Physiotherapists and occupational therapists need to build on
the principles of SRE for developing methods that are appropriate for
patients with deficient sensation and for patients with recovering sensation. In the next and final chapter, we shall suggest that there are also
wider applications for Sensory Re-education.

Chapter 10
Wider applications

The advocate of a novel therapy has to resist the temptation to offer it as a panacea. At the same time, sensory loss after stroke is not necessarily limited to the hand, and stroke is not the only condition which can disturb sensory function. This final chapter takes a brief look beyond the hands of stroke patients in order to see whether there are other areas for sensory re-education in stroke and in other categories of patients. Given the general neglect of sensory issues in rehabilitation, there is a dearth of research to build on, and conjecture rushes in to fill the gaps. Much of this chapter is therefore highly speculative, but this will be excusable if it generates new ways of looking at familiar conditions and new areas for research.

Sensory problems in standing and walking after stroke

Someone who has had a stroke can often be recognized from afar by the way he stands and walks. The characteristic features – the asymmetry of stance, the stiffness and jerkiness of gait – have been described and analysed by many authors (Perry, 1969; Knutsson and Richards, 1979; Dickstein, et al, 1984). Stroke patients who have sensory loss in the lower limb can also be recognized by their gait. Although it has features of the more typical 'spastic' hemiplegic gait, it tends to be less rigid, looser, more jerky – even 'ataxic' – and more varied, and to leave one in doubt about the diagnosis: could it be a peripheral neuropathy, multiple sclerosis or even that model of the insensate gait so seldom seen – tabes dorsalis? The fact that there is a sensory deficit in the lower limb tends to be overlooked when the patient is tested by stroking his shins with cotton wool, but it is at once apparent if his feet are tested for object recognition. Sitting with his feet a few centimetres above the floor, the patient will be unable to recognize common objects – a book, a tennis ball, a cup – placed under his affected foot, whereas he has no difficulty with his other foot. His sense of position – testing his toes, ankles and knees while he lies face down – is also likely to be severely disturbed. How does the sensory loss affect the patient's gait?

With the help of two colleagues and a pair of Kistler force plates for recording ground-reaction forces, I recorded the kinetics of gait in 20 hemiplegic patients, eight of them with marked sensory loss in the lower limb. The patients with sensory loss had force amplitudes very similar to those of the patients with intact sensation, but the *timing* of peak forces, particularly in the direction of walking, were strikingly different and deviated much more from normal gait (Yekutiel, Bar and Najenson, 1979). It would be interesting to repeat this study and, if the same results are observed, to explore the effects of sensory re-education on the timing of the kinetic events in their gait. Studies of the role of proprioception in stance and gait have yielded controversial results, and the subject needs pursuing.

Cerebral palsy

In cerebral palsy (CP), as in stroke, the motor impairment dominates both the clinical picture and the aims of therapy, and the possibility that there is also an invisible sensory impairment is seldom recognized. For years the subject suffered from a neglect sanctioned by the authoritative pronounce-ments of Osler and later of Freud to the effect that in CP 'sensation is not often disturbed' (Osler, 1889/1987). This view was finally challenged in the 1950s by Crothers, Tizard and Paine who re-examined several hundreds of CP patients whom they had seen as children during the preceding 20 years. In over 70% of those with hemiplegia they found sensory deficits (notably, astereognosis) which previous examinations had neither tested for nor diagnosed, and they suggested that poor sensation might account for the absence of functional improvement in a number of their patients who had undergone tendon transfers at the wrist (Tizard and Crothers, 1952; Tizard, Paine and Crothers, 1954). They also noted that underdevelopment of the hemiplegic hand and arm was more closely correlated with the existence of sensory impairment than with the motor severity.

This breakthrough was followed by a flurry of publications over the next ten years with authors reporting sensory deficit in up to 80% of children with spastic CP, prevalence being much lower in those with athetoid CP. This new interest at least highlighted the importance of good sensation as a prerequisite for surgery (Goldner and Ferlic, 1966), but it led to little else. Interest died down as quickly as it had sprung up, though two recent studies have helped to keep the subject from total neglect (Lesný et al., 1993; Yekutiel, Jariwala and Stretch, 1994).

Cerebral palsy seems to be at least as important as stroke as a target for exploring the effectiveness of SRE. Not only is sensory deficit disabling in its own right, but it must contribute to the CP child's motor disabilities. One would expect the phenomenon of 'learned non-use' to have a profound effect on the motor development of a child born with defective somatic sensation in one hand or one side of the body. However, the few comments that have been made about sensory deficit in CP – notably in hemiplegic children – have tended to see the sensory impairment as secondary to the motor impairment, owing its existence 'to the fact that the hand has never, by reason of its powerlessness, been used as a palpating organ' (Critchley, 1953). This echoes Déjérine's notion sixty years earlier of an 'astereognosis through inexperience' in what he called 'a virgin hand' (quoted by Crothers and Paine, 1959/1988). The assumption is that a child who has no voluntary use of his hand will never learn to feel with it, rather than that inadequate sensation will prevent a child using his hand. In a congenital condition it is difficult to attribute priority to either the sensory or the motor impairment, and the relation between sensory and motor function in children with CP is far from simple. Although astereognosis in the hand tends to be associated with poor hand function (Crothers and Paine, 1959/1988; Tachdjian and Minear, 1958), a paralysed hand does not necessarily lack sensation: there are children with perfect sensation in hands that are totally non-functional and that have never been used (Tachdjian and Minear, 1958; Monfraix, Tardieu and Tardieu, 1961; Yekutiel, 1996). Such children throw interesting light on the controversies surrounding the part that experience and learning play in the development of sensory perception. More relevant to the agenda of this book are the questions which they raise about the neurophysiology of sensory perception. In view of the well-documented plasticity of cortical maps and the existence of a 'cortical space race' (Katz, 1993), how is it that the sensory discriminative powers of these children's hands – in whatever way they came to be developed – have been retained in perfect condition in spite of a lifetime of disuse? The crucial role of activity in the development of the visual cortex has been recognized for decades, and in Chapter 4 we saw that there is now a large body of evidence, not only from manipulation of rat's whiskers or paws but from human studies, that the size of the somatosensory representation in the cortex is also profoundly affected by use and disuse. How are we to explain the development and retention of a perfectly functioning neural system which has never been used? This and many other unanswered questions make the subject of sensory perception in children with cerebral palsy a rich and little explored field for research.

Returning to the subject of sensory re-education in CP, Crothers and Paine wrote 40 years ago: 'the extent to which sensory perception ... could be improved by experience and practice has not been fully explored' (Crothers and Paine, 1959/1988). In the 1960s, the new interest in sensation in CP prompted some attempts at sensory training, with varying success. Monfraix and Tardieu (1961) published anecdotal descriptions of the successes and failures of a method they had introduced for re-educating 'manual perception'. Ferreri (1962) reported statistically significant improvement in stereognosis in eight young adults with CP after a few weeks of training, but Kenny (1966) failed to improve stereognosis in four children trained intensively for six months. The subject is still virtually virgin territory awaiting exploration. SRE, with its emphasis on interest and motivation and its easy transformation into games and play, would seem to be a good method for improving sensory function in children with cerebral palsy.

Other conditions

If, in stroke and in cerebral palsy, the examination of sensation is in the best cases perfunctory, in the worst simply not done, – and these are conditions with a known risk of sensory disturbance – it comes as no surprise that sensory deficits are seldom looked for in the general run of orthopaedics and traumatology. And yet, there are at least two ways in which trauma to the musculoskeletal system can produce sensory dysfunction which, if overlooked and untreated, can contribute to permanent disability.

The first is by direct damage to nerve fibres at the site of the injury. Doctors making a first examination of trauma patients almost invariably look out for gross involvement of the major nerves in the area, but there may be damage to nerve fibres which is hard to discern but of considerable importance to functional recovery. The best example of this comes from the fruitful collaboration of Freeman and Wyke in the 1960s on what they called the deafferentation of the ankle joint (Freeman and Wyke, 1964). In the laboratory, Wyke studied the articular receptors and nerves in the joint capsules and ligaments of animals' hind limbs and showed that these nerves, which mediate pain and awareness of joint position, also play a vital role in postural stabilization of the joint by reflex regulation of tone in the muscles that pass over it. Meanwhile, Freeman, an orthopaedic surgeon, was confronting the problem that 40% of ankle sprains leave the ankle in a state of 'functional instability': patients reported that the ankle tended to 'give way', and there was a high risk of repeated sprain. He could find no explanation in the clinical condition of the ankle. Wyke's work provided the clue: the afferent nerve fibres have a much lower tensile strength than the surrounding collagen fibres of the capsule and ligaments and are therefore the first structures to be torn when the ligaments are overstretched. Cutting articular nerve fibres in a cat caused the animal to walk unsteadily. Perhaps the problem in Freeman's patients was a proprioceptive deficit? This proved to be the answer. The large majority of patients immediately after ankle sprain showed great unsteadiness when trying to stand on the leg with eyes closed, and this was still evident one year later in those patients who developed functional instability (Freeman, Dean and Hanham, 1965). The final step was the demonstration that both the test of proprioception and the stability of the ankle were improved by exercising on a balance board rather than by the more traditional regime for strengthening muscles and increasing range of movement (Freeman, 1965). Freeman regarded the balancing exercises as a form of sensory retraining to meet the postural demands of everyday walking, including the unexpected perturbations which can lead to a sprained ankle. The nervous system learned (or developed new strategies) to answer postural challenges with the remaining systems at its disposal.

Most subsequent studies have supported Freeman's hypothesis. Repeated ankle sprain seems to cause not only poorer postural control but also decreased ability to detect passive movement at the ankle joint (Garn and Newton, 1988).

Wider applications

The second way in which musculoskeletal injuries can cause widespread disorders of sensorimotor function as well as localized motor dysfunction arises from the fact that every movement we make in our daily lives involves not only the 'prime mover' muscles directly responsible for the movement but also the recruitment of muscles all over the body – both in anticipation of the movement and while it is being carried out – to ensure postural stability. The anticipatory work of muscles in the legs, hips and trunk before a standing subject raises an arm was described long ago (Belen'kil, Gurfinkel and Pal'tsev, 1967), with a brief note to the effect that they are lost after a long period of bed rest. This and later studies (for instance, Horak et al., 1984) suggest that the delicate pattern of activity in widely dispersed muscles necessary for raising an arm (to comb one's hair or to wave to a friend) may be upset, not only by a period in hospital, but by a few weeks with a leg in plaster, a spell of backache or any of a multitude of apparently non-neurological mishaps. This recalls the work of Leont'ev and Zaporozhets (1945/1960) and their emphasis on the 'disco-ordination' phenomena almost universal in their patients with purely peripheral but severe musculoskeletal injuries. Recovery meant the restoration of the injured limb to its proper place in the patient's activity and self-perception, and they insisted that co-ordination must be re-established before attempting to improve range of joint movement or muscle strength. Perhaps the order of priority for physiotherapy in orthopaedic and trauma cases should be revised and listed as: sensation and co-ordination, then muscle strength, and last of all range of movement.

The book by Leont'ev and Zaporozhets makes exciting reading because they disregard many of the conceptual – one could say 'professional' – borders which transect the field of medicine in the West. They move with ease between orthopaedics, neurology and psychology and do not expect their patients' behaviour or problems to belong neatly to one or other category. Fodor, the title of whose book – 'The modularity of mind' – speaks for itself, wrote: 'The condition for successful science (in physics... as well as psychology) is that nature should have joints to carve it at: relatively simple subsystems which can be artificially isolated and which behave, in isolation, in something like the way that they behave *in situ*' (Fodor, 1983). However, it can also be illuminating to ignore the 'joints'. This grants a certain freedom to survey the scene as a whole and to see how it looks from a number of different viewpoints.

Conclusion

This book attempts to give a fresh look at the problems of stroke patients and at one aspect – a sensory one – that has been relatively neglected. The method of approaching it, by Sensory Rehabilitation, has as its basis the view that learning involves active mental processing (Howe, 1998) and that therapy for stroke patients needs to be active and interesting if it is to tap the brain's potential for functional reorganization. This principle is not limited to sensory function, but applies – as shown by the eclectic nature of its theoretical basis – to all aspects of recovery after stroke and, in all likelihood, to other areas of rehabilitation. If this principle were adopted and adhered to by all rehabilitation therapists, I believe that this could give birth to a new style of therapy, both more challenging to the recovering brain and more effective, perhaps demonstrably so. The outlook for stroke patients could only be improved.

References

Abercrombie MLJ, Lindon RL, Tyson M (1964) Associated movements in normal and physically handicapped children. Developmental Medicine and Child Neurology 6: 573–80.

Adams GF, Hurwitz LJ (1963) Mental barriers to recovery from strokes. Lancet 2: 533–7.

Adams RD, Victor M, Ropper AH (1997) Principles of Neurology. New York: McGraw-Hill.

Adey R, Noda H (1973) Influence of eye movements on geniculostriate excitability in the cat. Journal of Physiology London 235: 805–21.

Ahissar E, Vaadia E, Ahissar M, Bergman H, Arieli A et al. (1992) Dependence of cortical plasticity on correlated activity of single neurons and on behavioral context. Science 257: 1412–15.

Allport A (1993) Attention and control: have we been asking the wrong questions? A critical review of twenty-five years. In Meyer DE, Kornblum S (Eds) Attention and Performance XIV. Cambridge, Mass: MIT Press, pp. 210–18.

Anderson EK (1971) Sensory impairments in hemiplegia. Archives of Physical Medicine and Rehabilitation 52: 293–7.

Anderson EK, Choy E (1970) Parietal lobe syndromes in hemiplegia. American Journal of Occupational Therapy 24: 13–18.

Ashburn A (1995) A review of current physiotherapy in the management of stroke In Harrison MA (Ed.) Physiotherapy in Stroke Management. Edinburgh: Churchill Livingstone, pp. 3–22.

Ashburn A, Partridge C, De Souza L (1993) Physiotherapy in the rehabilitation of stroke: a review. Clinical Rehabilitation 7: 337–45.

Astrom M (1996) Generalized anxiety disorder in stroke patients. Stroke 27: 270–5.

Bach-y-Rita P (1986) Brain plasticity as a basis for therapeutic procedures. In Bach-y-Rita P (Ed.) Recovery of Function: Theoretical Considerations for Brain Injury Rehabilitation. Toronto: Huber Publishers, pp. 225–63.

Bandura A, Schunk D (1981) Cultivating competence, self-efficacy, and intrinsic interest through proximal self-motivation. Journal of Personality and Social Psychology 41: 586–98.

Barer DH (1990) The influence of visual and tactile inattention on predictions for recovery from acute stroke. Quarterly Journal of Medicine 273: 21–32.

Bastings EP, Rapisarda G, Pennisi G, de Noordhout AM, Lenaerts M et al. (1997) Mechanisms of hand motor recovery after stroke: an electrophysiologic study of central motor pathways. Journal of Neurologic Rehabilitation 11: 97–108.

Bateson G (1979) Mind and Nature: A Necessary Unity. London: Wildwood House.

Bell C (1833) The hand: its mechanism and vital endowments as evincing design. The Bridgewater Treatises, IV. London: William Pickering.

Belen'kil VY, Gurfinkel VS, Pal'tsev YI (1967) Elements of control of voluntary movements. Biofizika 12: 154–61.

Benecke R, Meyer B-U, Freund H-J (1991) Reorganization of descending motor pathways in patients after hemispherectomy and severe hemispheric lesions demonstrated by magnetic brain stimulation. Experimental Brain Research 83: 419–26.

Bergman L, van der Meulen JHP, Limburg M, Habbema JDF (1995) Costs of medical care after first-ever stroke in the Netherlands. Stroke 26: 1830–6.

Bernstein N (1967) The Co-ordination and Regulation of Movements. Oxford: Pergamon Press.

Bisiach E, Capitani E, Porta E (1985) Two basic properties of space representation in the brain: evidence from unilateral neglect. Journal of Neurology, Neurosurgery, and Psychiatry 48: 141–4.

Bisiach E, Vallar G, Perani D, Papagno C, Berti A (1986) Unawareness of disease following lesions of the right hemisphere: anosognosia for hemiplegia and anosognosia for hemianopia. Neuropsychologia 24: 471–82.

Bobath B (1970) Adult Hemiplegia: Evaluation and Treatment. London: Heinemann.

Bohannon RW, Horton MG, Wikholm JB (1991) Importance of four variables of walking to patients with stroke. International Journal of Rehabilitation Research 14: 246–50.

Bowsher D (1993) Sensory consequences of stroke. Lancet 341: 156.

Brain WR (1933) Diseases of the Nervous System. London: Oxford University Press.

Brain WR (1941) Visual disorientation with special reference to lesions of the right cerebral hemisphere. Brain 64: 244–72.

Braune S, Schady W (1993) Changes in sensation after nerve injury or amputation: the role of central factors. Journal of Neurology, Neurosurgery, and Psychiatry 56: 393–9.

Broadbent DE (1958) Perception and Communication. London: Pergamon Press.

Brodal A (1973) Self-observations and neuro-anatomical considerations after a stroke. Brain 96: 675–94.

Bromley DB (1966) The Psychology of Human Ageing. Harmondsworth, UK: Penguin Books.

Brunnstrom S (1970) Movement Therapy in Hemiplegia. London: Harper and Row.

Bulman RJ, Wortman CB (1977) Attribution of blame and coping in the real world: severe accident victims react to their lot. Journal of Personality and Social Psychology 35: 351–63.

Burke D (1988) Spasticity as an adaptation to pyramidal tract injury. Advances in Neurology 47: 401–23.

Burton H, Macleod AK, Videen TO, Raichle ME (1997) Multiple foci in parietal and frontal cortex activated by rubbing embossed grating patterns across fingerpads: a positron emission tomography study in humans. Cerebral Cortex 7: 3–17.

Cairns J (1997) Matters of Life and Death: Perspectives on Public Health, Molecular Biology, Cancer, and the Prospects for the Human Race. Princeton, NJ: Princeton University Press.

Calford MB, Tweedale R (1990) Interhemispheric transfer of plasticity in the cerebral cortex. Science 249: 805–7.

Caramia MD, Iani C, Bernardi G (1996) Cerebral plasticity after stroke as revealed by ipsilateral responses to magnetic stimulation. NeuroReport 7: 1756–60.

Carey LM (1995) Somatosensory loss after stroke. Critical Reviews in Physical and Rehabilitation Medicine 7: 51–91.

Carey LM, Matyas TA, Oke LE (1990) Facilitation of sensory rehabilitation using a discriminative training programme with stroke patients. Proceedings of the World Federation of Occupational Therapists 10th International Congress, Melbourne.

Carey LM, Matyas TA, Oke LE (1993) Sensory loss in stroke patients: effective tactile and proprioceptive discrimination training. Archives of Physical Medicine and Rehabilitation 74: 602–11.

Carey LM, Oke LE, Matyas TA (1996) Impaired limb position after stroke: a quantitative test for clinical use. Archives of Physical Medicine and Rehabilitation 77: 1271–8.

Carmon A (1971) Disturbances of tactile sensitivity in patients with unilateral cerebral lesions. Cortex 7: 83–97.

Carr J, Shepherd R (1982) A Motor Relearning Programme for Stroke. London: William Heinemann.

Castillo S, Starkstein SE, Fedoroff P, Price TR, Robinson RG (1993) Generalized anxiety after stroke. Journal of Nervous and Mental Disease 181: 100–6.

Cernacek J (1961) Contralateral motor irradiation – cerebral dominance. Archives of Neurology 4: 165–72.

Chao LL, Knight RT (1997) Prefrontal deficits in attention and inhibitory control with aging. Cerebral Cortex 7: 63–9.

Chapin JK, Woodward DJ (1982) Somatic sensory transmission to the cortex during movement: gating of single cell responses to touch. Experimental Neurology 78: 654–69.

Chapman CE (1994) Active versus passive touch: factors influencing the transmission of somatosensory signals to primary somatosensory cortex. Canadian Journal of Physiology and Pharmacology 72: 558–70.

Charpentier A (1891) Analyse expérimentale de quelques éléments de la sensation des poids. (Experimental study of some aspects of weight perception). Archives de Physiologie Normales et Pathologiques 3: 122–35.

Cherry EC (1957) On Human Communication: A Review, a Survey, and a Criticism. New York: John Wiley.

Chester CS, McLaren CE (1989) Somatosensory evoked response and recovery from stroke. Archives of Physical Medicine and Rehabilitation 70: 520–5.

Chiou IL, Burnett CN (1985) Values of activities of daily living: a survey of stroke patients and their home therapists. Physical Therapy 65: 901–6.

Chollett F, Di Piero V, Wise RJS, Brooks J, Dolan RJ et al. (1991) The functional anatomy of motor recovery after stroke in humans: a study with Positron Emission Tomography. Annals of Neurology 29: 63–71.

Chollett F, Weiller C. (1994) Imaging recovery of function following brain injury. Current Opinion in Neurobiology 4: 226–30.

Cohen LG, Brasil-Neto JP, Pascual-Leone A, Hallett M (1993) Plasticity of cortical motor output organization following deafferentation, cerebral lesions, and skill acquisition. Advances in Neurology 63: 187–200.

Condon C, Weinberger NM (1991) Habituation produces frequency-specific plasticity of receptive fields in auditory cortex. Behavioral Neuroscience 105: 416–30.

Cope KJ (1991) Grasp force control in older adults. Journal of Motor Behavior 23: 251–8.

Cotton E, Kinsman R (1983) Conductive Education and Adult Hemiplegia. Edinburgh: Churchill Livingstone.

Coulter JD (1974) Sensory transmission through leminiscal pathway during voluntary movement in the cat. Journal of Neurophysiology 37: 831–45.

Craig JC (1992) Anomalous sensations following prolonged tactile stimulation. Neuropsychologia 31: 277–91.

Craske B (1977) Perception of impossible limb positions induced by tendon vibration. Science 196: 71–3.

Critchley M (1949) The phenomenon of tactile inattention with special reference to parietal lesions. Brain 72: 538–61.

Critchley M (1953) Tactile thought, with special reference to the blind. Brain 76: 19–35.

Crothers B, Paine RS (1959/1988) The Natural History of Cerebral Palsy. London: MacKeith.

Cruikshank SJ, Weinberger NM (1996) Evidence for the Hebbian hypothesis in experience-dependent physiological plasticity of neocortex: a critical review. Brain Research Reviews 22: 191–228.

Dannenbaum RM, Dykes RW (1988) Sensory loss in the hand after sensory stroke: therapeutic rationale. Archives of Physical Medicine and Rehabilitation 69: 833–9.

Dannenbaum RM, Dykes RW (1990) Evaluating sustained touch-pressure in severe sensory deficits: meeting an unanswered need. Archives of Physical Medicine and Rehabilitation 71: 455–9.

Dannenbaum RM, Jones LA (1993) The assessment and treatment of patients who have sensory loss following cortical lesions. Journal of Hand Therapy 6: 130–8.

Dean CM, Shepherd RB (1997) Task-related training improves performance of seated reaching tasks after stroke. Stroke 28: 722–8.

Dellon AL (1988) Evaluation of Sensibility and Re-education of Sensation in the Hand. Baltimore MD: Lucas Printing Company.

Denny-Brown D (1966) The organistic (holistic) approach: the neurological impact of Kurt Goldstein. Neuropsychologia 4: 293–7.

Denny-Brown D, Chambers RA (1958) The parietal lobes and behaviour. Research Publications of the Association for Research in Mental Diseases 36: 35–116.

Desrosiers J, Bourbonnais D, Bravo G, Roy PM, Guay M (1996) Performance of the 'unaffected' extremity of elderly stroke patients. Stroke 27: 1564–70.

Deutsch JA, Deutsch D (1963) Attention: some theoretical considerations. Psychological Review 70: 80–90.

Devor M, Schonfeld D, Seltzer Z, Wall PD (1979) Two modes of cutaneous reinervation following nerve injury. Journal of Comparative Neurology 185: 211–20.

Dickstein R, Nissan M, Pillar T, Scheer D (1984) Foot-ground pressure pattern of standing hemiplegic patients: major characteristics and pattern of improvement. Physical Therapy 64: 19–23.

Dittmar CM, Gliner JA (1987) Bilateral hand performance with divided attention after a cerebral vascular accident. American Journal of Occupational Therapy 41: 96–101.

Dorman PJ, Sandercock PAG (1996) Considerations in the design of clinical trials of neuroprotective therapy in acute stroke. Stroke 27: 1509–15.

Driver J (1994) Unilateral neglect and normal attention. Neuropsychological Rehabilitation 4: 123–6.

Dykes RW (1997) Mechanisms controlling neuronal plasticity in somatosensory cortex. Canadian Journal of Physiology and Pharmacology 75: 535–45.

Edin BB, Abbs JH (1991) Finger movement responses of cutaneous mechanoreceptors in the dorsal skin of the human hand. Journal of Neurophysiology 65: 657–70.

Edmans JA, Towle D, Lincoln NB (1991) The recovery of perceptual problems after stroke and the impact on daily life. Clinical Rehabilitation 5: 301–9.

Eisenstein EM, Carlson AD (1997) A comparative approach to the behavior called 'learned helplessness'. Behavioural Brain Research 86: 149–60.

Elbert T, Pantev C, Wienbruch C, Rockstroh B, Taub E (1995) Increased cortical representation of the fingers of the left hand in string players. Science 270: 305–7.

Elliott T, Howarth CI, Shadbolt NR (1996) Axonal processes and neural plasticity. II: Adult somatosensory maps. Cerebral Cortex 6: 789–93.

Ernst E (1990) A review of stroke rehabilitation and physiotherapy. Stroke 211: 1081-5.

Eysenck MW, Keane MT (1990) Cognitive Psychology: A Student's Handbook. London: Erlbaum.

Faggin BM, Nguyen KT, Nicolelis MAL (1997) Immediate and simultaneous sensory reorganization at cortical and subcortical levels of the somatosensory system. Proceedings of the National Academy of Sciences of the United States of America 94: 9428–33.

Fazeli S, Collingridge GL (1997) Cortical Plasticity. Oxford: Oxford University Press.

Feather N (1982) Expectations and Actions: Expectancy-value Models in Psychology. Hillsdale, NJ: Erlbaum.

Feibel JH, Berk S, Joynt RJ (1979) The unmet needs of stroke survivors. Neurology 29: 592.

Feigenson JS (1979) Stroke rehabilitation: effectiveness, benefits, and cost: some practical considerations. Stroke 10: 1–4.

Feinberg TE, Rothi LJG, Heilman KM (1986) Multimodal agnosia after unilateral hemisphere lesion. Neurology 36: 864–7.

Feine JS, Chapman CE, Lund JP, Duncan GH, Bushnell MC (1990) The perception of painful and nonpainful stimuli during voluntary motor activity in man. Somatosensory and Motor Research 7: 113–24.

Ferreri JA (1962) Intensive stereognostic training: effect on spastic cerebral palsied adults. American Journal of Occupational Therapy 16: 141–2.

Fisher CM (1992) Concerning the mechanism of recovery in stroke hemiplegia. Canadian Journal of Neurological Sciences 19: 57–63.

Fitts PM, Posner MI (1967) Human Performance. California. Brooks/Cole.

Fodor JA (1983) The Modularity of Mind. Cambridge, Mass: MIT Press.

Folstein MF, Maiberger R, McHugh PR (1977) Mood disorder as a specific complication of stroke. Journal of Neurology, Neurosurgery, and Psychiatry 40: 1018–20.

Forster FM, Shields CD (1959) Cortical sensory defects causing disability. Archives of Physical Medicine and Rehabilitation 40: 56–61.

Freeman MAR (1965) Coordination exercises in the treatment of functional instability of the foot. Physiotherapy 51: 393–5.

Freeman MAR, Dean MRE, Hanham IWF (1965) The etiology and prevention of functional instability of the foot. Journal of Bone and Joint Surgery 47: 678–85.

Freeman MAR, Wyke BD (1964) The innervation of the cat's knee joint. Journal of Anatomy 98: 299–300.

Fugl-Meyer AR, Lääskö L, Leyman I, Olsson S, Steglind S (1975) The post-stroke hemiplegic patient: I. A method for evaluation of physical performance. Scandinavian Journal of Rehabilitation Medicine 7: 13–31.

Garn SN, Newton RA (1988) Kinesthetic awareness in subjects with multiple ankle sprains. Physical Therapy 68: 1667–71.

Garraghty PE, Kaas JH (1991) Functional reorganization in adult monkey thalamus after peripheral nerve injury. NeuroReport 2: 747–50.

Garraway WM, Whisnant JP (1987) The changing pattern of hypertension and the declining incidence of stroke. Journal of the American Medical Association 258: 214–7.

Garraway WM, Whisnant JP, Drury I (1983) The changing pattern of survival following stroke. Stroke 14: 699–703.

Garraway WM, Whisnant JP, Kurland LT, O'Fallon WM (1979) Changing pattern of cerebral infarction: 1945–1974. Stroke 10: 657–63.

Gerstmann J (1940) Syndrome of finger agnosia, disorientation for right and left, agraphia and acalculalia. Archives of Neurology and Psychiatry 44: 398–408.

Ghez C, Pisa M (1972) Inhibition of afferent transmission in cuneate nucleus during voluntary movement in the cat. Brain Research 40: 145–51.

Gibson JJ (1962) Observations on active touch. Psychological Review 69: 477–91.

Gibson JJ (1966) The Senses Considered as Perceptual Systems. Boston: Houghton Mifflin Company.

Gilbert P (1992) Depression: The Evolution of Powerlessness. Hove, UK: Erlbaum.

Glees P (1986) Functional cerebral reorganization following hemispherectomy in man and after small experimental lesions in primates. In Bach-y-Rita P (Ed.) Recovery of Function: Theoretical Considerations for Brain Injury Rehabilitation. Toronto: Huber Publishers, pp. 106–26.

Glover J, Corkhill A (1987) Influence of paraphrased repetitions on the spacing effect. Journal of Educational Psychology 79: 198–9.

Goff B (1969) Appropriate afferent stimulation. Physiotherapy 55: 9–17.

Goffman E (1961) Asylums: Essays on the Social Situation of Mental Patients and Other Inmates. New York: Doubleday.

Goldman H (1966) Improvement of double simultaneous stimulation perception in hemiplegic patients. Archives of Physical Medicine and Rehabilitation 47: 681–7.

Goldner JF, Ferlic DC (1966) Sensory status of the hand as related to reconstructive surgery of the upper extremity in cerebral palsy. Clinical Orthopaedics 46: 87–92.

Good TL, Brophy JE (1990) Educational Psychology: A Realistic Approach. 4th edition. New York: Longman.

Goodale MA, Milner AD (1992) Separate visual paths for perception and action. Trends in Neurosciences 15: 20–5.

Goodstein RK (1983) Overview: cerebrovascular accident and the hospitalized elderly – a multidimensional clinical problem. American Journal of Psychiatry 140: 141–7.

Goodwin GM, McCloskey DI, Matthews PBC (1972) The contribution of muscle afferents to kinaesthesia shown by vibration-induced illusions of movement and by the effects of paralysing joint afferents. Brain 95: 705–48.

Gottlieb D, Kipnis M, Sister E, Medvedev V, Brill S et al. (1997) Classification of stroke rehabilitation patients with a simple impairment scale. Journal of Neurologic Rehabilitation 11: 239–43.

Green JB (1967) An electromyographic study of mirror movements. Neurology 17: 91–4.

Gregory RL (1961) The brain as an engineering problem. In Thorpe WH, Zangwill OL (Eds) Current Problems in Animal Behaviour. Cambridge: Cambridge University Press, pp. 307–30.

Griffith H, Davidson M (1966) Long-term changes in intellect and behavior after hemispherectomy. Journal of Neurology, Neurosurgery, and Psychiatry 29: 571–6.

Griffith VE (1980) Observations on patients dysphasic after stroke. British Medical Journal 281: 1608–9.

Grotta J, Bratina P (1995) Subjective experiences of 24 patients dramatically recovering from stroke. Stroke 26 :1285–8.

Haaland KY, Vranes LF, Goodwin JS, Garry PJ (1987) Wisconsin card sort test performance in a healthy elderly population. Journal of Gerontology 39: 166–9.

Hale LA, Eales CJ (1998) Recovery of walking function in stroke patients after minimal rehabilitation. Physiotherapy Research International 3: 194–205.

Hallin RG, Wiesenfeld Z, Lindblom U (1981) Neurophysiological studies of patients with sutured median nerves: faulty sensory localization after nerve regeneration and its physiological correlates. Experimental Neurology 73: 90–106.

Halnan CRE, Wright GH (1960) Tactile localization. Brain 83: 677–700.

Hanger HC, Sainsbury R (1996) Sensory abnormalities after stroke. Stroke 27: 1439.

Hankey GJ, Jamrozik K, Broadhurst RJ, Forbes S, Burvill P et al. (1998) Long-term risk of first recurrent stroke in the Perth community study. Stroke 29: 2491–500.

Head H (1918) Sensation and the cerebral cortex. Brain 41: 57–253.

Healy C, LeQuesne P, Lynn B (1996) Collateral sprouting of cutaneous nerves in man. Brain 119: 2063–72.

Hill AB (1962) Statistical Methods in Clinical and Preventive Medicine. London: Livingstone.

Hill K, Ellis P, Bernhard J, Maggs P, Hull S (1997) Balance and mobility outcomes for stroke patients: a comprehensive audit. Australian Journal of Physiotherapy 43: 173–9.

Holmes G (1927) Disorders of sensation produced by cortical lesions. Brain 50: 413–27.

Honoré J, Bourdeaud'hui M, Sparrow L (1989) Reduction of cutaneous reaction time by directing eyes towards the source of stimulation. Neuropsychologia 27: 367–71.

Horak FB, Esselman P, Anderson ME Lynch MK (1984) The effects of movement velocity, mass displaced, and task certainty on associated postural adjustments made by normal and hemiplegic individuals. Journal of Neurology, Neurosurgery, and Psychiatry 47: 1020–8.

Horch KW (1979) Guidance of regrowing sensory axons after cutaneous nerve lesions in the cat. Journal of Neurophysiology 42: 1437–49.

House A, Dennis M, Mogridge L, Warlow C, Hawton K et al. (1991) Mood disorders in the year after first stroke. British Journal of Psychiatry 158: 83–92.

House A, Dennis M, Molyneux A, Warlow C, Hawton K (1989) Emotionalism after stroke. British Medical Journal 298: 991–4.

Howe MJA (1998) Principles of Abilities and Human Learning. Hove, UK: Psychology Press.

Hsaio SS, O'Shaughnessy DM, Johnson KO (1993) Effects of selective attention on spatial form processing in monkey primary and secondary somatosensory cortex. Journal of Neurophysiology 70: 444–7.

Humphrey T (1964) Some correlations between the appearance of human fetal reflexes and the development of the nervous system. Progress in Brain Research 4: 93–133.

Huskisson EC (1974) Measurement of pain. Lancet 2: 1127–31.

Huttunen J, Wikstrom H, Korvenoja A, Seppalainen AM, Aronen H et al. (1996) Significance of the second somatosensory cortex in sensorimotor integration: enhancement of sensory responses during finger movements. NeuroReport 7: 1009–12.

Hyvarinen J, Poranen A, Jokinen Y (1980) Influence of attentive behavior on neuronal responses to vibration in primary somatosensory cortex of the monkey. Journal of Neurophysiology 43: 870–82.

Inbal R, Rousso M, Ashur H, Wall PD, Devor M (1987) Collateral sprouting in skin and sensory recovery after nerve injury in man. Pain 28: 141–54.

Indredavik B, Bakke F, Solberg R, Rokseth R, Haaheim LL et al. (1991) Benefit of a stroke unit: a randomized controlled trial. Stroke 22: 1026–31.

Isaacs B (1978) Problems and solutions in rehabilitation of stroke patients. Geriatrics 33: 87–91.

Iwamura Y, Iriki A, Tanaka M (1994) Bilateral hand representation in the postcentral somatosensory cortex. Nature 369: 554–6.

James W (1890) The Principles of Psychology. New York: Holt.

Jeannerod M, Michel F, Prablanc C (1984) The control of hand movements in a case of hemianaesthesia following a parietal lesion. Brain 107: 899–920.

Jenkins WM, Merzenich MM (1987) Reorganization of neocortical representations after brain injury: a neurophysiological model of the bases of recovery from stroke. Progress in Brain Research 71: 249–66.

Jenkins WM, Merzenich MM, Ochs MT, Allard T, Guic-Rables E (1990) Functional reorganization of primary somatosensory cortex in adult owl monkeys after behaviorally controlled tactile stimulation. Journal of Neurophysiology 63: 82–104.

Jiang W, Lamarre Y, Chapman CE (1990) Modulation of cutaneous cortical evoked potentials during isometric and isotonic contractions in the monkey. Brain Research 536: 69–78.

Johansson BB (1996) Functional outcome in rats transferred to an enriched environment 15 days after focal brain ischemia. Stroke 27: 324–6.

Johansson RS (1996) Sensory control of dexterous manipulation in humans. In Wing AM, Haggard P, Flanagan JR (Eds) Hand and Brain: The Neurophysiology and Psychology of Hand Movements. San Diego, California: Academic Press, pp. 381–414.

Johnston M, Gilbert P, Partridge C, Collins J (1992) Changing perceived control in patients with physical disabilities: an intervention study with patients receiving rehabilitation. British Journal of Clinical Psychology 31: 89–94.

Jones EG, Powell TPS (1969) Connexions of the somatic sensory cortex of the rhesus monkey. II Contralateral cortical connexions. Brain 92: 717–30.

Jones RD, Donaldson IM, Parkin PJ (1989) Impairment and recovery of ipsilateral sensory-motor function following unilateral cerebral infarction. Brain 112: 113–32.

Kaas JH (1991) Plasticity of sensory and motor maps in adult animals. Annual Review of Neuroscience 14: 137–67.

Kaas JH, Nelson RJ, Sur M, Lin CS, Merzenich MM (1979) Multiple representations of the body within the primary somatosensory cortex of primates. Science 204: 521–3.

Kaplan RM, Atkins CJ, Reinsch S (1984) Specific efficacy expectations mediate exercise compliance in patients with COPD. Health Psychology 2: 223–42.

Karp E, Belmont I, Birch HG (1971) Delayed sensory-motor processing following cerebral damage. Cortex 7: 417–25.

Kase CS, Wolf PA, Kelly-Hayes M, Kannel WB, Beiser A et al. (1998) Intellectual decline after stroke: the Framingham study. Stroke 29: 805–12.

Katz D (1925/1989) The World of Touch (translated by LE Krueger). Hillside, New Jersey: Erlbaum.

Katz LC (1993) Cortical space race. Nature 364: 578–9.

Kelly-Hayes M (1990) Time intervals, survival, and destination: three crucial variables in stroke outcome research. Stroke 21 (suppl. II): 24–6.

Kelly-Hayes M, Wolf PA, Kase CS, Gresham GE, Kannel WB et al. (1989) Time course of functional recovery after stroke: the Framingham study. Journal of Neurologic Rehabilitation 3: 65–70.

Kelman HR, Willner A (1962) Problems in measurement and evaluation of rehabilitation. Archives of Physical Medicine and Rehabilitation 43: 172–81.

Kelso JAS, Holt KG, Flatt AE (1980) The role of proprioception in the perception and control of human movement: towards a theoretical reassessment. Perception and Psychophysics 28: 45–52.

Kennedy F (1924) Astereognosis. Archives of Neurology and Psychiatry 12: 305–7.

Kenny WE (1966) The importance of sensori-perceptuo-agnosia in the examination, the understanding and the management of cerebral palsy. Clinical Orthopaedics 46: 45–52.

Kidd G, Lawes N, Musa I (1992) Understanding Neuroplasticity: A Basis for Clinical Rehabilitation. London: Edward Arnold.

Kim JS (1992) Pure sensory stroke: clinical-radiological correlates of 21 cases. Stroke 23: 983–7.

Kim JS, Choi-Kwon S (1996) Discriminative sensory dysfunction after unilateral stroke. Stroke 27: 677–82.

Kinsbourne M (1977) Hemineglect and hemisphere rivalry. Advances in Neurology 18: 41–9.

Klag NJ, Whelton PK, Seidler AJ (1989) Decline in US stroke mortality: demographic trends and antihypertensive treatment. Stroke 20: 14–21.

Klatzky RL, Lederman SJ (1987) The intelligent hand. The Psychology of Learning and Motivation 21: 121–51.

Klatzky RL, Lederman SJ, Metzger V (1985) Identifying objects by touch: an 'expert system.' Perception and Psychophysics 37: 299–302.

Klopfer PH (1992) Structure and function in the CNS. Behavioral and Brain Sciences 15: 281.

Knott M, Voss D (1968) Proprioceptive Muscular Facilitation. New York: Harper and Row.

Knutsson E, Richards C (1979) Different types of disturbed motor control in gait of hemiparetic patients. Brain 102: 405–30.

Koerber HR, Mirnics K (1996) Plasticity of dorsal horn cell receptive fields after peripheral nerve regeneration. Journal of Neurophysiology 75; 2255–67.

Koerber HR, Seymour AW, Mendell LM (1989) Mismatches between peripheral receptor type and central projections after peripheral nerve regeneration. Neuroscience Letters 99: 67–72.

Konno Y (1989) Changes of body sensation through muscular relaxation, using the method of measuring two-point limen (in Japanese). Shinrigaku-Kenkyu 60: 209–15.

Krueger WCF (1929) The effect of overlearning on retention. Journal of Experimental Psychology 12: 71–8.

Kusoffsky A, Wadell I, Nilsson BY (1982) The relationship between sensory impairment and motor recovery in patients with hemiplegia. Scandinavian Journal of Rehabilitation Medicine 14: 27–32.

Kwakkel G, Kollen BJ, Wagenaar RC (1999) Therapy impact on functional recovery in stroke rehabilitation. Physiotherapy 85: 377–91.

Lackner JR (1988) Some proprioceptive influences on the perceptual representation of body shape and orientation. Brain 111: 281–97.

La Joie WL, Reddy NM, Melvin JL (1982) Somatosensory evoked potentials: their predictive value in right hemiplegia. Archives of Physical Medicine and Rehabilitation 63: 223–6.

Langhorne P, Williams BO, Gilchrist W, Howle K (1993) Do stroke units save lives? Lancet 342: 395.

Langton Hewer R (1990) Rehabilitation after stroke. Quarterly Journal of Medicine 76: 659–74.

Langton Hewer R (1993) The epidemiology of disabling neurological disorders. In: Greenwood R, Barnes MP, McMillan TM, et al. (Eds) Neurological Rehabilitation. London: Churchill Livingstone, pp. 3–12.

Lapin L (1975) Statistics: Meaning and Method. New York: Harcourt.

Larmande P, Cambier J (1981) Influence de l'état d'activation hémisphérique sur le phénomène d'extinction sensitive chez 10 patients atteints de lésions hémisphériques droites. Revue Neurologique 137: 285–90.

Lazarus JAC, Todor JI (1987) Age differences in the magnitude of associated movement. Developmental Medicine and Child Neurology 29: 726–33.

Lederman SJ, Klatzky RL (1990) Haptic classification of common objects: knowledge-driven exploration. Cognitive Psychology 22: 421–59.

Lee RG, van Donkelaar P (1995) Mechanisms underlying functional recovery following stroke. Canadian Journal of Neurological Sciences 22: 257–63.

Leont'ev AN, Zaporozhets AV (1945/1960) Rehabilitation of Hand Function (translated by Basil Haig). London: Pergamon Press.

Lesný I, Stehlik A, Tomášek J, Tománková A Havliček I (1993) Sensory disorders in cerebral palsy: two-point discrimination. Developmental Medicine and Child Neurology 35: 402–405.

LeVere ND, LeVere TE (1982) Recovery of function after brain damage: support for the compensation theory of the behavioural deficit. Physiological Psychology 10: 165–74.

Levine DN (1990) Unawareness of visual and sensorimotor defects: a hypothesis. Brain and Cognition 13: 233–81.

Lincoln NB, Crow JL, Jackson JM, Waters GR, Adams SA et al. (1991) The unreliability of sensory assessments. Clinical Rehabilitation 5: 273–82.

Lincoln NB, Willis D, Philips SA, Juby LC, Berman P (1996) Comparison of rehabilitation practice on hospital wards for stroke patients. Stroke 27: 18–23.

Livingstone WK (1947) Evidence of active invasion of denervated areas by sensory fibers from neighboring nerves in man. Journal of Neurosurgery 4: 140–63.

Locke EA, Latham GP (1984) Goal setting: A Motivational Technique That Works. Englewood Cliffs, N.J: Prentice-Hall.

Luria AR (1963) Restoration of Function after Brain Injury. Oxford: Pergamon Press.

MacHale SM, O'Rourke SJ, Wardlow JM, Dennis MS (1998) Depression and its relation to lesion location after stroke. Journal of Neurology, Neurosurgery, and Psychiatry 64: 371–4.

Mahler H (1975) Health – demystification and medical technology. Lancet 2: 829–33.

Marr D (1976) Early processing of visual information. Philosophical Transactions of the Royal Society, London, B, 275: 483–524.

Marsden CD, Rothwell JC, Day BL (1984) The use of peripheral feedback in the control of movement. Trends in Neurosciences 7: 253–7.

Marshall JC, Halligan PW, Robertson IH (1993) Contemporary theories of unilateral neglect: a critical review. In Robertson IH and Marshall JC (Eds) Unilateral Neglect: Clinical and Experimental Studies. Hove UK: Erlbaum, pp. 311–29.

Marshall RN, Jennings LS (1990) Performance objectives in the stance phase of human pathological walking. Human Movement Science 9: 599–611.

Marshall SC, Grinnell D, Heisel B, Newall A, Hunt L (1997) Attentional deficits in stroke patients: a visual dual task experiment. Archives of Physical Medicine and Rehabilitation 78: 7–12.

Maslow AH (1954) Motivation and Personality. New York: Harper and Row.

Mathiowetz V, Bass-Haugen J (1994) Motor behavior research: implications for therapeutic approaches to central nervous system dysfunction. American Journal of Occupational Therapy 48: 733–45.

Mattingley JB, Driver J, Beschin N, Robertson IH (1997) Attentional competition between modalities: extinction between touch and vision after right hemisphere damage. Neuropsychologia 35: 867–80.

Mauguière F, Desmedt JE, Courjon J (1983) Astereognosis and dissociated loss of frontal or parietal components of somatosensory evoked potentials in hemispheric lesions. Brain 106: 271–311.

McGuire M, Troisi A (1998) Darwinian Psychiatry. Oxford: Oxford University Press.

Merzenich MM, Jenkins WM (1993) Reorganization of cortical representations of the hand following alterations of skin inputs induced by nerve injury, skin island transfers, and experience. Journal of Hand Therapy 6: 89–104.

Merzenich MM, Kaas JH (1982) Reorganization of mammalian somatosensory cortex following peripheral nerve injury. Trends in Neurosciences 5: 434–6.

Mesulam MM (1981) A cortical network for directed attention and unilateral neglect. Annals of Neurology 10: 309–25.

Mesulam MM (1994) The multiplicity of neglect phenomena. Neuropsychological rehabilitation. 4: 173–6.

Moberg E (1964) Aspects of sensation in reconstructive surgery of the upper extremity. Journal of Bone and Joint Surgery 46A: 817–25.

Moberg E (1983) The role of cutaneous afferents in position sense, kinaesthesia, and motor function of the hand. Brain 106: 1–19.

Monfraix C, Tardieu G (1961) Development of manual perception in the child with cerebral palsy during re-education. Cerebral Palsy Bulletin 3: 553–8.

Monfraix C, Tardieu G, Tardieu C (1961) Disturbances of manual perception in children with cerebral palsy. Cerebral Palsy Bulletin 3: 544–52.

Moscovitch M, Behrmann M (1994) Coding of spatial information in the somatosensory system: evidence from patients with neglect following parietal lobe damage. Journal of Cognitive Neuroscience 6: 151–5.

Moskowitz E, Lightbody FEH, Freitag NS (1972) Long term follow-up of the poststroke patient. Archives of Physical Medicine and Rehabilitation 53: 167–73.

Motomura N, Yamadori A, Asaba H, Sakai T, Sawada T (1990) Failure to manipulate objects secondary to active touch disturbance. Cortex: 26: 473–7.

Mountcastle VB (1975) The view from within: pathways to the study of perception. Johns Hopkins Medical Journal 136: 109–31.

Mulder T (1991) A process-oriented model of human motor behavior: towards a theory-based rehabilitation approach. Physical Therapy 71: 157–64.

Nakayama H, Jørgensen HS, Raaschou HO, Olsen TS (1994) Recovery of upper extremity function in stroke patients: the Copenhagen stroke study. Archives of Physical Medicine and Rehabilitation 75: 394–8.

Nathan P (1997) The Nervous System. 4th edn. London: Whurr.

Neisser U (1967) Cognitive Psychology. Englewood Cliffs, NJ: Prentice-Hall.

Nudo RJ, Wise BM, SiFuentes F, Milliken GW (1996) Neural substrates for the effects of rehabilitative training on motor recovery after ischemic infarct. Science 272: 1791–4.

Oatley K, Boulton W (1985) A social theory of depression in reaction to life events. Psychological Review 92: 372–88.

Ohlsson AL, Johansson BB (1995) Environment influences functional outcome of cerebral infarction in rats. Stroke 26: 644–9.

Olsen TS (1989) Improvement of function and motor impairment after stroke. Journal of Neurologic Rehabilitation 3:187–92.

Osler W (1889/1987) The Cerebral Palsies of Children. London: Mac Keith Press.

Palmer E, Ashby P, Hajek VE (1992) Ipsilateral fast corticospinal pathways do not account for recovery in stroke. Annals of Neurology 32: 519–25.

Papakostopoulos D, Cooper R, Crow HJ (1975) Inhibition of cortical evoked potentials and sensation by self-initiated movement in man. Nature 258: 321–3.

Parker VM, Wade DT, Langton Hewer R (1986) Loss of arm function after stroke: measurement, frequency, and recovery. International Rehabilitation Medicine 8: 69–73.

Partridge CJ (1984) Recovery from conditions involving physical disability. Physiotherapy 70: 233–5.

Partridge C, Johnston M (1989) Perceived control of recovery from physical disability: measurement and prediction. British Journal of Clinical Psychology 28: 53–9.

Partridge CJ, de Weerdt W (1995) Different approaches to physiotherapy in stroke. Reviews in Clinical Gerontology 5: 199–209.

Pascual-Leone A, Cammarota A, Wassermann EM, Brasil-Neto JP, Cohen LG et al. (1993) Modulation of motor cortical outputs to the reading hand of Braille readers. Annals of Neurology 34: 33–7.

Pascual-Leone A, Dang N, Cohen LG, Brasil-Neto JP, Cammarota A et al. (1995) Modulation of muscle responses evoked by transcranial magnetic stimulation during the acquisition of new fine motor skills. Journal of Neurophysiology 74: 1037–45.

Pascual-Leone A, Grafman J, Hallett M (1994) Modulation of cortical motor output maps during development of implicit and explicit knowledge. Science 263: 1287–92.

Pascual-Leone A, Torres F (1993) Plasticity of the sensorimotor cortex representation of the reading finger in Braille readers. Brain 116: 39–52.

Paterson A, Zangwill OL (1944) Disorders of visual space perception associated with lesions of the right cerebral hemisphere. Brain 67: 331–58.

Pause M, Kunesch E, Binkofski F, Freund H-J (1989) Sensorimotor disturbances in patients with lesions of the parietal cortex. Brain 112: 1599–625.

Paykel ES (1978) Contribution of life events to causation of psychiatric illness. Psychological Medicine 8: 245–53.

Payton OD, Ozer MN, Nelson CE (1990) Patient Participation in Program Planning: A Manual for Therapists. Philadelphia: F.A.Davis Company.

Pedersen PM, Jørgensen HS, Nakayama H, Raaschou HO, Olsen TS (1996) Frequency, determinants, and consequences of anosognosia in acute stroke. Journal of Neurologic Rehabilitation 10: 243–50.

Penfield W, Boldrey E (1937) Somatic and motor sensory representation in the cerebral cortex of man as studied by electrical stimulation. Brain 60: 389–443.

Perry J (1969) The mechanics of walking in hemiplegia. Clinical Orthopaedics and Related Research 63: 23–31.

Phillips CG (1986) Movements of the Hand: The Sherrington Lectures XVII. Liverpool: Liverpool University Press.

Pierson JM, Bradshaw JL, Meyer TF, Howard MJ, Bradshaw JA (1991) Direction of gaze during vibrotactile choice reaction time tasks. Neuropsychologia 29: 925–8.

Posner MI, Boies SW (1971) Components of attention. Psychological Review 78: 391–408.

Posner MI, Rafal RD (1987) Cognitive theories of attention and the rehabilitation of attentional deficits. In Meier MJ, Benton AL, Diller L (Eds) Neuropsychological Rehabilitation. Edinburgh: Churchill Livingstone.

Rabbitt PMA (1965) An age decrement in the ability to ignore irrelevant information. Journal of Gerontology 20: 233–8.

Rasmusson DD (1982) Reorganization of raccoon somatosensory cortex following removal of the fifth digit. Journal of Comparative Neurology 205: 313–26.

Rasmusson DD (1996) Changes in the response properties of neurons in the ventroposterior lateral thalamic nucleus of the raccoon after peripheral deafferentation. Journal of Neurophysiology 75: 2441–50.

Recanzone GH, Merzenich MM, Jenkins WM (1992a) Frequency discrimination training engaging a restricted skin surface results in an emergence of a cutaneous response zone in cortical area 3a. Journal of Neurophysiology 67: 1057–70.

Recanzone GH, Merzenich MM, Jenkins WM, Grajski KA, Dinse HR (1992b) Topographic reorganization of the hand representation in cortical area 3b of owl monkeys trained in a frequency-discrimination task. Journal of Neurophysiology 67: 1031–56.

Recanzone GH, Merzenich MM, Shreiner CE (1992c) Changes in the distributed temporal response properties of SI cortical neurons reflect improvements in performance on a temporally based tactile discrimination task. Journal of Neurophysiology 67: 1071–91.

Reding MJ (1990) A model stroke classification scheme and its use in outcome research. Stroke 21(suppl. II): 35–7.

Reed CL (1994) Perceptual dependence for shape and texture during haptic processing. Perception 23: 349–66.

Reed CL, Caselli RJ, Farah MJ (1996) Tactile agnosia: underlying impairment and implications for normal object recognition. Brain 119: 875–88.

Reid A, Chesson R (1998) Goal attainment scaling: is it appropriate for stroke patients and their physiotherapists? Physiotherapy 84: 136–144.

Riggs LA, Ratcliff F, Cornsweet JC, Cornsweet TN (1953) The disappearance of steadily fixated objects. Journal of the Optical Society of America 43: 495–501.

Rivers WHR, Head H (1908) A human experiment in nerve division. Brain 31: 323–450.

Robertson SL, Jones LA (1994) Tactile sensory impairments and prehensile function in subjects with left-hemisphere cerebral lesions. Archives of Physical Medicine and Rehabilitation 75: 1108–117.

Robinson RG, Price TR (1982) Post-stroke depressive disorders: a follow-up study of 103 patients. Stroke 13: 635–641.

Roland PE (1992) Somatosensory detection of microgeometry, macrogeometry and kinesthesia after localized lesions of the cerebral hemispheres in man. Brain Research Reviews 12: 43–94.

Roll JP, Gilhodes JC (1995) Proprioceptive sensory codes mediating movement trajectory perception: human hand vibration-induced drawing illusions. Canadian Journal of Physiology and Pharmacology 73: 295–304.

Rose L, Bakal DA, Fung TS, Farn P, Weaver LE (1994) Tactile extinction and functional status after stroke. Stroke 25: 1973–6.

Rosenzweig MR, Bennett EL (1996) Psychobiology of plasticity: effects of training and experience on brain and behavior. Behavioural Brain Research 78: 57–65.

Rosenzweig MR, Bennett EL, Diamond MC (1972) Brain changes in response to experience. Scientific American 226(2): 22–29.

Rothwell JC, Traub MM, Day BL, Obeso JA, Thomas PK et al. (1982) Manual motor performance in a deafferented man. Brain 105: 515–42.

Rotter J (1966) Generalized expectancies for internal versus external control of reinforcement. Psychological Monographs 80: 1–28.

Ruch TC, Fulton JF, German WJ (1938) Sensory discrimination in monkeys, chimpanzee and man after lesions of the parietal lobe. Archives of Neurology and Psychiatry 39: 919–38.

Rushton DN, Rothwell JC, Craggs MD (1981) Gating of somatosensory evoked potentials during different kinds of movement in man. Brain 104: 465–91.

Ryle G (1949) The Concept of Mind. London: Hutchinson

Sacks O (1984) A Leg to Stand on. New York: Summit Books.

Sadato N, Pascual-Leone A, Grafman J, Ibanez V, Deiber MP et al. (1996) Activation of the primary visual cortex by Braille reading in blind subjects. Nature 380: 526–8.

Sadka M (1972) Perceptual problems in neurology. Australian Journal of Physiotherapy 18: 37–42.

Sainburg RL, Poizner H, Ghez C (1993) Loss of proprioception produces deficits in interjoint coordination. Journal of Neurophysiology 70: 2136–47.

Sathian K, Zangaladze A (1997) Tactile learning is task specific but transfers between fingers. Perception and Psychophysics 59: 119–128.

Schwartz AB (1994) Direct cortical representation of drawing. Science 265: 540–2.

Seligman MEP (1975) Helplessness: On Depression Development and Death. San Francisco: Freeman and Co.

Semmes J (1965) A non-tactual factor in astereognosis. Neuropsychologia 3: 295–315.

Shadish WR, Hickman D, Arvick MC (1981) Psychological problems of spinal cord injury patients: emotional distress as a function of time and locus of control. Journal of Consulting and Clinical Psychology 49: 297–305.

Shah S (1989) Admissions, patterns of utilization and dispositions of cases of acute stroke in Brisbane hospitals. Medical Journal of Australia 150: 256–60.

Sheikh K, Brennan PJ, Meade TW, Smith DS, Goldenberg E (1983) Predictors of mortality and disability in stroke. Journal of Epidemiology and Community Health 37: 70–4.

Shepherd R, Carr J (1991) An emergent or dynamical systems view of movement dysfunction. Australian Journal of Physiotherapy 31: 4–5.

Sherrington CS (1906) The Integrative Action of the Nervous System. New Haven: Yale University Press.

Silvestrini M, Caltagirone C, Cupini LM, Matteis M, Troisi E et al. (1993) Activation of healthy hemisphere in post-stroke recovery: a transcranial doppler study. Stroke 24: 1673–7.

Smith DL, Akhtar AJ, Garraway WM (1983) Proprioceptive and spatial neglect after stroke. Age and Ageing 12: 63–9.

Smith S, Rothkopf E (1984) Contextual enrichment and distribution of practice in the classroom. Cognition and Instruction 1: 341–58.

Starkstein SE, Cohen BS, Fedoroff P, Parikh RM, Price TR et al. (1990) Relationship between anxiety disorders and depressive disorders in patients with cerebrovascular injury. Archives of General Psychiatry 47: 246–51.

Steinberg FU (1973) The stroke registry: a prospective method of studying stroke. Archives of Physical Medicine and Rehabilitation 54: 31–5.

Stern PH, McDowell F, Miller JM, Robinson M (1971) Factors influencing stroke rehabilitation. Stroke 2: 213–18.

Stone SP, Wilson B, Wroot A, Halligan PW, Lange LS et al.(1991) The assessment of visuospatial neglect after acute stroke. Journal of Neurology, Neurosurgery, and Psychiatry 54: 345–50

Stroemer RP, Kent TA, Hulsebosch CE (1995) Neocortical neural sprouting, synaptogenesis, and behavioral recovery after neocortical infarction in rats. Stroke 26: 2135–44.

Stroke Unit Trialists' Collaboration (1997) Collaborative systematic review of the randomised trials of organised inpatient (stroke unit) care after stroke. British Medical Journal 314: 1151–9.

Sullivan R (1969) Experimentally induced somatagnosia. Archives of General Psychiatry 20: 71–7.

Sumner AJ (1990) Aberrant reinnervation. Muscle and Nerve 13: 801–3.

Sutherling WW, Levesque MF, Baumgartner C (1992) Cortical sensory representation of the human hand: size of finger regions and non-overlapping digit somatotopy. Neurology 42: 1020–8.

Tachdjian MO, Minear WL (1958) Sensory disturbances in the hands of children with cerebral palsy. Journal of Bone and Joint Surgery 40A: 85–90.

Tatemichi TK, Desmond DW, Stern Y, Paik M, Sano M et al. (1994) Cognitive impairments after stroke: frequency, patterns, and relationship to functional activities. Journal of Neurology, Neurosurgery, and Psychiatry 57: 202–7.

Taub E (1980) Somatosensory deafferentation research with monkeys: implications for rehabilitation medicine. In Ince LP (Ed.) Behavioral Psychology in Rehabilitation Medicine: Clinical Applications. Baltimore: Williams and Wilkins.

Taylor DP (1974) Treatment goals for quadriplegic and paraplegic patients. American Journal of Occupational Therapy 28: 22–9.

Taylor MM, Schaeffer JN, Blumenthal FS, Grisell JL (1971) Perceptual training in patients with left hemiplegia. Archives of Physical Medicine and Rehabilitation 52: 163–9.

Taylor TN, Davis PH, Torner JC, Holmes J, Meyer JW et al. (1996) Lifetime cost of stroke in the United States. Stroke 27: 1459–66.

Teasell RW, Gillen M (1993) Upper extremity disorders and pain following stroke. Physical Medicine and Rehabilitation 7: 133–46.

Tegner R (1988) Tactile sensibility in parietal lesions. Journal of Neurology, Neurosurgery, and Psychiatry 52: 669–70.

Thomas C, Altenmuller E, Marckmann G, Kahrs J, Dichgans J (1997) Language processing in aphasia: changes in lateralization patterns during recovery reflect cerebral plasticity in adults. Electroencephalography and Clinical Neurophysiology 102: 86–9.

Tinson DJ (1989) How stroke patients spend their days. International Disability Studies 11: 45–9.

Tizard JPM, Crothers B (1952) Sensory disturbances in hemiplegia in childhood. Transactions of the American Neurological Association 77: 227–9.

Tizard JPM, Paine RS, Crothers B (1954) Disturbances of sensation in children with hemiplegia. Journal of the American Medical Association 155: 628–32.

Tomasello F, Mariani F, Fieschi C, Argentino C, Bono G et al. (1982) Assessment of inter-observer differences in the Italian multicenter study on reversible cerebral ischemia. Stroke 13: 32–5.

Traversa R, Cicinelli P, Bassi A, Rossini PM, Bernardi G (1997) Mapping of motor cortical reorganization after stroke: a brain stimulation study with focal magnetic pulses. Stroke 28: 110–17.

Treisman A (1969) Strategies and models of selective attention. Psychological Review 76: 282–99.

Tuomilehto J, Nuottimaki T, Salmi K, Aho K, Kotila M et al. (1995) Psychosocial and health status in stroke survivors after 14 years. Stroke 26: 971–5.

Twomey L (1996) The 'real' world of physiotherapy research. Editorial. Physiotherapy Theory and Practice 12: 65–6.

Ungerlieder CG, Mishkin M (1982) Two cortical visual systems. In Ingle J, Goodale MA, Mansfield RJW, (Eds) Analysis of Visual Behavior. Cambridge, Mass: MIT Press.

Vallar G, Sandroni P, Rusconi ML, Barbieri S (1991) Hemianopia, hemianesthesia, and spatial neglect. Neurology 41: 1918–22.

Van Buskirk C, Webster D (1955) Prognostic value of sensory defect in rehabilitation of hemiplegics. Neurology 5: 407–11.

Van Deusen Fox J (1964) Cutaneous stimulation: effects on selected tests of perception. American Journal of Occupational Therapy 18: 53–5.

Van Ravensberg CD, Tyldesley DA, Rozendal RH, Whiting HTA (1984) Visual perception in hemiplegic patients. Archives of Physical Medicine and Rehabilitation 65: 304–9.

Vega-Bermudez F, Johnson KO, Hsiao SS (1991) Human tactile pattern recognition: active versus passive touch, velocity effects, and patterns of confusion. Journal of Neurophysiology 65: 531–46.

Vinograd A, Taylor E, Grossman S (1962) Sensory retraining of the hemiplegic hand. American Journal of Occupational Therapy 16: 246–50.

Wade DT (1989) Measuring arm impairment and disability after stroke. International Disability Studies 11: 89–92.

Wade DT, Collen FM, Robb GF, Warlow CP (1992) Physiotherapy intervention late after stroke and mobility. British Medical Journal 304: 609–13.

Wade DT, Langton Hewer R, Skilbeck CE, David RM (1985) Stroke: A Critical Approach to Diagnosis, Treatment and Management. London: Chapman and Hall.

Wade DT, Legh-Smith J, Hewer RA (1987) Depressed mood after stroke: a community study of its frequency. British Journal of Psychiatry 151: 200–5.

Wade DT, Skilbeck CE, Langton Hewer R, Wood VA (1984) Therapy after stroke: amounts, determinants and effects. International Rehabilitation Medicine 6: 105–11.

Wade DT, Wood VA, Langton Hewer R (1985) Recovery after stroke: the first 3 months. Journal of Neurology, Neurosurgery, and Psychiatry 48: 7–13.

Wall JT, Kaas JH, Sur M, Nelson RJ, Felleman DJ et al. (1986) Functional reorganization in somatosensory cortical areas 3b and 1 of adult monkeys after median nerve repair: possible relationships to sensory recovery in humans. Journal of Neuroscience 6: 218–233.

Walsh RN (1981) Effects of environmental complexity and deprivation on brain anatomy and histology: a review. International Journal of Neuroscience 12: 33–51.

Walshe FMR (1923) On certain tonic or postural reflexes in hemiplegia, with special reference to the so-called 'associated movements'. Brain 46: 2–37.

Weber EH (1834/1978) De Tactu (The Sense of Touch) (translated by Ross HE). New York: Academic Press.

Webster N. (1966) Third International Dictionary. New York: Merriam Co.

Weddell G, Guttmann L, Gutmann E (1941) The local extension of nerve fibres into denervated areas of skin. Journal of Neurology, Neurosurgery, and Psychiatry 4: 206–25.

Weder B, Knorr U, Herzog H, Nebeling B, Kleinschmidt A et al. (1994) Tactile exploration of shape after subcortical ischaemic infarction studied with PET. Brain 117: 593–605.

Weiller C, Chollet F, Friston KJ, Wise RJS, Frackowiak RSJ (1992) Functional reorganization of the brain in recovery from striatocapsular infarction in man. Annals of Neurology 31: 463–72.

Weiller C, Ramsay SC, Wise RJS, Friston KJ, Frackowiak RSJ (1993) Individual patterns of functional reorganization in the human cerebral cortex after capsular infarction. Annals of Neurology 33: 181–9.

Weinberg J, Diller L, Gordon WA, Gerstman LJ, Lieberman A, et al. (1977) Visual scanning training effect on reading-related tasks in acquired right brain damage. Archives of Physical Medicine and Rehabilitation 58: 479–86.

Weinberg J, Diller L, Gordon WA, Gerstman LJ, Lieberman A, et al. (1979) Training sensory awareness and spatial organization in people with right brain damage. Archives of Physical Medicine and Rehabilitation 60: 491–6.

Weiner B (1966) The role of success and failure in the learning of easy and complex tasks. Journal of Personality and Social Psychology 3: 339–43.

Weiner B (1986) An Attributional Theory of Motivation and Emotion. New York: Springer-Verlag.

Westing G, Johansson RS (1984) Factors influencing the force control during precision grip. Experimental Brain Research 53: 277–84.

White, EL (1989) Cortical Circuits. Boston: Birkhauser.

Wilkinson PR, Wolfe CDA, Warburton FG, Rudd AG, Howard RS et al. (1997) A long-term follow-up of stroke patients. Stroke 28: 507–12.

Williams JM (1976) Synaesthetic adjectives: a possible law of semantic change. Language 52: 461–78.

Wolf SL, Lecraw DE, Barton LA, Jann BB (1989) Forced use of hemiplegic upper extremities to reverse the effect of learned nonuse among chronic stroke and head-injured patients. Experimental Neurology 104: 125–32.

Wolff PH, Gunnoe CE, Cohen C (1983) Associated movements as a measure of developmental age. Developmental Medicine and Child Neurology 25: 417–29.

World Health Organization (1971) Cerebrovascular diseases: prevention, treatment, and rehabilitation. WHO Technical Report Series 469: 1–57.

World Health Organization (1980) International classification of impairments, disabilities and handicaps: a manual of classification relating to the consequences of disease. Geneva: World Health Organization.

Wynn Parry CB (1973) Rehabilitation of the Hand. 3rd edn. London: Butterworths.

Wynn Parry CB, Salter M (1976) Sensory re-education after median nerve lesions. Hand 8: 250–7.

Yekutiel M (1977) Sensory re-education of the hand (in Hebrew). Israel Journal of Physiotherapy 26: 26–39.

Yekutiel M (1996) Hand sensation in children with cerebral palsy. Proceedings of the 1st Mediterranean Congress of Physical Medicine and Rehabilitation. Herzliya, Israel.

Yekutiel M, Bar A, Najenson T (1979) The amplitude and timing of peak ground forces in the gait of hemiplegic patients. Paper presented at the Combined Meeting of the 12th International Conference on Medical and Biological Engineering and the 5th International Conference on Medical Physics, Jerusalem.

Yekutiel M, Guttman E (1993) A controlled trial of the retraining of the sensory function of the hand in stroke patients. Journal of Neurology, Neurosurgery, and Psychiatry 56: 241–4.

Yekutiel M, Jariwala M, Stretch P (1994) Sensory deficit in the hands of children with cerebral palsy: a new look at assessment and prevalence. Developmental Medicine and Child Neurology 36: 619–24.

Yekutiel M, Robin GC, Yarom R (1981) Proprioceptive function in children with adolescent idiopathic scoliosis. Spine 6: 560–6.

Zeman BD, Yiannikas C (1989) Functional prognosis in stroke: use of somatosensory evoked potentials. Journal of Neurology, Neurosurgery, and Psychiatry 52: 242–7.

Index